learning to care for the aged

charlotte epstein

Temple University

learning to care for the aged

Reston Publishing Company, Inc., *A Prentice-Hall Company*

Reston, Virginia

Library of Congress Cataloging in Publication Data

Epstein, Charlotte.
    Learning to care for the aged.

    Bibliography: p.
    Includes index.
    1. Geriatric nursing—Study and teaching. I. Title.
[DNLM: 1. Geriatric nursing. 2. Nurse—Patient
relations. WY152 E64L]
RC954.E67   610.73′65   76-56458
ISBN 0-87909-442-7
ISBN 0-87909-441-9

10   9   8   7   6   5   4   3   2   1

Printed in the United States of America

to my father, my touchstone

contents

preface

No one knows better than a nurse that scientific knowledge does not guarantee effective professional functioning. An individual may know his anatomy and pharmacology, he may be adept at differential diagnosis, yet he may frighten the very young, cause the aged to be disheartened, and contribute to the feelings of isolation of the dying.

Nurses as a profession have for some time been involved in that area of professional education that goes beyond medical expertise and encourages the development of self-awareness, sensitivity to the needs of others, and skill in interacting productively. This book attempts to provide nurses with material that will facilitate continued development of awareness, sensitivity, and skill—especially in their relationships with old people.

Our national heritage bequeaths us prejudice and discrimination, and our individual life situations reinforce in us stereotypic thinking. Although some people forever complain that the schools are being forced to assume responsibility for what the home and the church should teach, schools have not ever dealt seriously with these problems. Still, many of us, despite the default of home and school, value people of different races, champion the rights of the young, and maintain communication and productive interaction across age lines.

But there are those of us who live in the adult world as if there were
no human races but our own, and no age groups with the good sense that
we have. For these adults, pupils are merely subjects for testing, Black
people are objects that cause anxiety, and aged patients are senile. For
these adults, the principles of action and interaction learned from textbooks, the statistics about groups, the lists of rules, and the careful
definitions never can break through the preconceptions and stereotypes.
For them, the principles applied never seem to work, and following the
rules becomes an exercise in futility. For them, children or other races
or old people do not become warm, three-dimensional, irritating, lovable,
perplexing human beings.

Even those of us who seem pretty free of the constraints of stereotyping and prejudices are often surprised to discover in our own thinking errors and misconceptions on which we are basing our decisions and
attempting our communications: Old people are conservative and rigid;
therefore, old people should be forced out of key decision–making positions if we are to make progress as an institution and as a nation. Old
people prefer to associate with people their own age; therefore, assign
them to room together and to live together. Old people are concerned
mainly with their children and grandchildren; therefore, don't talk to
them about politics or sex.

Errors of this kind increase the psychological distance between old
people and people of other ages, and deprive the younger among us of at
least one important benefit of cross-age association: the aged among us
can help us to accept the continuity of life, and to become a part of that
continuity with comfort. Benjamin Franklin wrote, "An old man in a
house is a good sign." Without the reassurance that the old can provide,
we stand on the edge of a precipice, afraid to look down on the darkness
of our own futures.

Unless we die young, old age is inevitable. It can be a good time
for us when we come to it, but only if we make it a good time for those
who are there now. The answer lies largely in the willingness to enter
upon a process of fostering communication, the ultimate result of which
is the ability to see every person as unique, with an essential dignity
that is a function of his own conception of self.

It is hoped that the exercises here will help this process of communication.

Perhaps a word of explanation is needed about a less tangible aspect
of the book—its tempo. The reader may notice that the background material, primarily found in the odd-numbered chapters, is a combination
of research findings, opinions of administrators and other workers in the
field of aging, and the experiences of ordinary people who are involved
in their personal lives with aged relatives and friends. Although this

combination may present a feeling of unevenness that requires abrupt shifting of gears in reading, it is an unevenness that I deliberately emphasize to make a point about knowledge of old age and aging: while the scientific data accumulate, and the administrators of programs and agencies struggle to implement public policy that is often in conflict with the data, people are living their lives with each other, making decisions, searching for ways to make their own aging and old age productive and meaningful. Nurses who enter the lives of people at various times of stress need to know that neither science nor public policy is giving most of us much help in making something good of our relationships with old people, and something good of our own old age. If a nurse is to intervene at appropriate points to introduce new knowledge and model new behavior, she must be sensitive to the existence of tensions associated with old age and cross-age interaction and be able to recognize the underlying prejudices of so many of those tensions. It is only by examining her own experiences, and then participating, first vicariously and then actually, in experiences with many old people and their families that the nurse can become a resource for her patients who are struggling to survive in an atmosphere of ambivalence and prejudice.

The intermingling of formal and informal data here, then, is designed to point out the intellectual and practical gaps in our approach to aging, and to help the nurse begin to close those gaps.

CHARLOTTE EPSTEIN

learning to care for the aged

1

*attitudes and behaviors
toward aging and the aged*

ambivalence

The Problem at All Levels

Donald Kent, Director of the Office of Aging, of the U.S. Department of Health, Education, and Welfare, several years ago told the National Conference of State Executives on Aging [1]:

> Inconsistencies [in our country] are rampant. On the one hand we are sure that individuals can never submit to the indignity of a means test for medical care but feel they can do so for housing. We are sure that older people want to be kept in the mainstream of life and equally true that we should be creating activity centers geared to a specific age group. We are sure that older people want to be independent and have many conferences on how to provide services and do things for them. We profess that we should never talk down to the aged and then proceed to design programs that would be patronizing to a 13-year-old. We advocate an income approach to meeting needs and spend much time developing programs of reduced fares, food, stamps, and other devices that erode the income principle.

Bernice Neugarten, speaking at the 9th Congress of Gerontology in Kiev, U.S.S.R., in 1972 voiced a concern that seems more universal than just one in our own country [2]:

> Social scientists are asking if generational conflicts are even now increasing in modern societies and if so, are they appearing in both directions—on the one hand, between the young and society at large; and on the other hand, between the old and society at large. Is a new age-divisiveness appearing and new antagonisms that can be called age-ism? Is the world entering a period of social change in which, like earlier struggles for political and economic rights, it is now also a struggle for age rights? If so, will the struggle be joined not only by the young but also by the old who might otherwise become its victims? . . .
> Anger toward the old may . . . be on the rise.

Although the phrasing of the concern is cautious, Neugarten sees rather hard evidence in the United States that the aged are already a cohort of victims: "Covert antagonisms toward the old are seen in the United States in the small percentage of the welfare dollar spent for services to the aged; by the pervasive pattern of attitudes that make Americans slow in providing meaningful roles for older people; even by the fact that research on aging is so slow to develop in both the biological and social sciences."

She looks for reasons for the rise in antagonism toward the old: "A growing proportion of power positions in the judiciary, the legislative, the business, and the professional arenas are occupied by older people, and because of seniority privileges among workers, the young and middle-aged become resentful. [A]s the number of retired increases, the economic burden is perceived as falling more and more on the middle-aged taxpayer."

She goes on to wonder what will happen in the future, with the almost inevitable rise in the population of older people:

> It is being said by at least a few biologists that a breakthrough [in discovering the factors that underlie the rate of aging] will occur within the next 20 years . . . and that . . . man will have . . . an additional 25 years of life. . . . If we are indeed facing a sudden new extension of the life-span, with a dramatic new increase in the proportions of the old, will industrialized societies be more ready than before, and be better prepared?
> The problems will be enormous.

But she points out that research evidence continues to chip away at our stereotypes. The implication is that old age, too, may reap the advantages of changes in our attitudes and our behaviors:

> Man's desire for longevity can now, if anything, be whetted by the findings of social scientists: for example, that the institutional arrangements of industrialized societies do not inevitably lead to the social isolation of the old; that man does not lose his ability to learn as he grows old; that there is no universal set of personality changes that lead inevitably to disengagement from society—in short, the old person stands to benefit as much from social advances as does the young person.

The conflicts between scientific data and feelings toward the old, between professed concern and practical neglect, are inevitably—on another level—transmitted to the children. Children reared in our culture get conflicting messages about age and old people, because the teachers of the young generally have not reconciled their own contradictory attitudes. Even Margaret Mead reveals evidence of such contradiction in her own life. She writes, "My paternal grandmother, who lived with us from the time my parents married until she died in 1927 . . . was the most decisive influence in my life." [3]

"I think it was my grandmother who gave me my ease in being a woman." But she remembers, "Mother never ceased to resent the fact that Grandma lived with us. . . ." [4]

She believes strongly that grandparents are important to the full development of the child: "Children ought to have a chance to enjoy their grandparents." [5] However, I have been unable to find anywhere in her writings that she believes in making the old person an integral part of the nuclear family. Her plea for the care of children by the family has no analogue in her writings about the aged.

She worries that "A society imperils its own future when, out of negligence or contempt, it overlooks the need of children to be reared in a family . . . or when, in the midst of plenty, some families cannot give their children adequate food and shelter, safe activity and rest." [6] But she seems to see no danger to a society that "out of negligence or contempt" prevents *the aged* from being comfortably included in the family.

Although she is clear about the ambivalence toward old people that children are exposed to, she does not go beyond her commitment to the two-generation nuclear family and see the possibility of a need for grandparents in the same house. Is it the echo of her mother's resentment that restrains her? [7]

> Young parents often tell me how essential it is for children to have grandparents who are close to them. Yet in most American homes there are two tones of voice for visits to and from grandparents. The children's voices are expected to ring with joy and expectancy and the parents speak of such visits with anxiety or resignation. The differences between generations have been so great in this country of immigrants, continual mobility and rapid change that many parents and their grown-up children are desperately uneasy with each other.

Margaret Mead has become for many of us the twentieth-century renaissance woman. Her articulate descriptions of contemporary life are fearlessly critical, but the love and faith in an improvable humanity that permeates them saves her readers from that destructive cynicism that prevents action for change. But when she says, "The integrity of the society rests with the integrity of family life," [8] she is talking only about the nuclear family. She believes that grandparents give grandchildren a sense of continuity and an awareness of the reality of history. She herself is inextricably linked to the grandmother she lived with in childhood: "The closest friends I have made all through life," she says, "have been people who also grew up close to a loved and loving grandmother or grandfather." [9] But perhaps the most widely-listened-to observer of life today makes no very strong statement about the value of extending the nuclear family to include the aged.

The evidence of ambivalence toward the aged is everywhere. While a government agency proposes desperately needed housing for the elderly, citizens in the same community engage in what one writer described as a "middle-aged riot" in protest against that housing. Through it all, many of the participants reiterate that they have nothing against old people. "Age-ism reflects a deep-seated uneasiness on the part of the young and middle-aged—a personal revulsion to and distaste for growing old, disease, disability; and fear of powerlessness, 'uselessness,' and death." [10]

A physician writes a generally sensitive book about caring for aged parents, but at the outset he makes it perfectly clear that the aged parent must not be permitted to upset his adult child's home. He advises an offspring, "You cannot make it your home *and* somebody else's. It can't be your living room and your father's. When Father moves in with you, he is a member of the family but he must accept your rules and regulations even if he doesn't agree with them. That is the price he must be willing to pay." [11]

In many families, one adult offspring often takes on the responsibility for caring for an aged parent, while the other adult children live with guilt for not doing for their parent what they vaguely feel they ought to be doing. This guilt seems pervasive in our society. It manifests itself in erratic behaviors, vis-à-vis the aged, of politicians and scientists, professionals, and just family members.

One form this guilt/ambivalence takes is in the response to other adults who have taken aged parents into their homes. The adult who suddenly is living with an aged parent becomes conditioned to refraining from mentioning any difficulty she is having in dealing with the situation. When she wonders aloud how she is to arrange to attend an important professional meeting because she must prepare and serve dinner to someone who will go hungry if she does not, the usual response, given in a mock-loving voice and served up with a sweetly martyred smile is, "Just remember, when they're gone, then it's too late."

When she complains that the tax laws provide for all kinds of entertainment for businessmen, but will give no help to people to take on the support of aged parents, even her accountant says matter-of-factly, "At least you have him with you."

So she is forever left with the feeling that she is somehow ungrateful for saying anything at all about having a problem. She has assumed the responsibility voluntarily, she loves her father and does everything to make him comfortable, she changes her style of life and even the outward manifestations of her personality, but she is permitted to say nothing, except that she loves the whole idea.

Bear in mind that this pressure to button up is maintained not by people who are themselves caring for parents. I do not have the evidence, but I would hazard a guess that they are generally those who have managed to avoid the responsibility. They are, however, often people who have had a parent die not long ago. Perhaps their advice is a concession to the guilt they have been unable to unload.

These kinds of pressures to keep feelings hidden and to refrain from revealing the realities of an interpersonal situation counter the trend in this country toward more and more analysis of relationships and greater candor in communication.

The dear soul who has managed to waste her own life by spending it all on attending her own mother until she died now purrs and coos at other adults caring for a parent, "I think you're doing a wonderful thing. You're a *good* person." But she is an anachronism, openly commended but secretly held in contempt, and in some ways, an object of fear as an example of what can happen to the middle-aged adult in a society that has not resolved its conflicts about the aged.

Even the responses of professionals to those who are caring for the aged—without preparation or societal guidelines—are curiously contradictory, or often seemingly colored by what appears to be firm resolve to ignore the reality and deal in platitudes and stereotypes. There is the physiatrist who persists in assuming that adults who have aged parents at home do little besides administer to those parents. He indulges in little homilies like, "Walking is very important. If he's sitting and watching television, get him to stand up and walk around the house every hour. Walk with him if he doesn't think of it himself. Walking is very good for you, too." Every hour on the hour!

This physiatrist is the same person who recommends that a nursing home is the best place for an aged parent, because he will be lonely at home alone during the day when the rest of the family is out working. He does not seem very clear about where he stands, even in a specific situation. Is the family to spend *all* its time caring for the aged, or *none* of its time?

Those who must spend much of their time with old people are often cold, uncaring, impatient, and, sometimes, downright cruel. Yet I have seen adults who encounter a small, bent, white-haired old man walking purposefully along, *smile* at the companion with that saccharine grimace that says, "Isn't that *sweet?*" They may even actually say that *aloud,* as if the old man were a cute infant, or a cuddly dog being walked. He is a *conversation piece!* A pet!

This is similar to the behavior that enrages some black people who are victimized by an apparent contradiction in responses. The white people who coo and cluck over black babies are usually the same ones who are hostile toward black adults. The whites are at a loss to understand the coolness or downright unfriendliness with which their overtures to a child are met.

The question arises: Are those who think an old man is *sweet* the same ones who refuse to permit the building of homes for old people in their neighborhoods?

Ambivalence and Communication

The ambivalence toward the aged may well be at least partly a function of the difficulties of communication between parents and off-spring generally. Nor am I talking about a "generation gap." Actually, I believe the generation gap to be a myth manufactured to explain the defective communication between parents and children, between younger people and older people. This fact becomes readily apparent when one examines the quality of communication between individuals in the *same* generation. The differences are hardly apparent.

The outstanding characteristic of communication—or the lack of it—between individuals in the same or different generations is that they simply do not listen to each other.

Here is a transcript of a conversation between two five-year-olds:
"Will you come to my house after school?"
"My brother is coming home."
"After school?"
"He's in college."
And you should hear these two participating in a group discussion! One of them gets started on the story of her life and never stops for breath. Her eyes turn inward and she relives every moment as she speaks. She is completely out of touch with any of the other children or the teacher, all of whom keep trying unsuccessfully to interrupt her flow of words. Sometimes the other one gets the first word in, and she is off and running. She does give some of the others a chance to say something every once in a while, but then she immediately picks up her narrative or starts a new one as if they had never spoken.

And here is a conversation between two octogenarians:
"I think you're absolutely right. The city administration ought to be impeached!"
"The mayor's not bad. It's just one or two of the boys in the back room who keep trying to run the show."
"I know you always said we shouldn't vote for any of them, but what was the alternative?"
"I've often wondered if a politician really has any power or is only the messenger boy of the people behind the scenes who pay the bills."
"Well, there isn't much point in crying over spilt milk. What's done is done."

Listen to two 40-year-olds:

"Joanie is doing so well in school. I'm really very proud of her."

"I wonder what college Mary will finally decide on."

"One day she's going to be a doctor. That delicate little thing!"

"It's so difficult to find exactly the right one. The wrong choice can be a hindrance to her for the rest of her life."

"Would you go to a woman doctor?"

"That reminds me—my doctor said to be sure and avoid peaches. He seems to think it's peaches that are causing that rash right here."

Now hear a 25-year-old mother and her five-year-old son:

"You like school, don't you dear?"

"Johnnie wouldn't play with me."

"School is not the place to play. You should be working hard and doing what the teacher tells you to do."

"His brother wouldn't let him."

"What did you learn in school today?"

"Do you think I could have a dog like Johnnie?"

And here we have a 35-year-old and a 75-year-old:

"Mrs. Walter, I want you to eat raw carrots and celery. They're good for you. They counteract some of the side effects of the medicine you're taking."

"Doctor, do you think it would be all right if I took that pill in the afternoon—so I could sleep in the morning?"

"The pills cause a little constipation, so you need the roughage."

"I really hate being wakened every morning just to take a pill."

"That's right. You take the pills faithfully and you'll find that the tremors almost disappear."

You see, it isn't a *generation* gap that we have; it's a gap between people. The egocentricity of our near-infancy never really develops into adequate awareness of and interaction with others. Each of us goes through life frustrated at being inadequately understood. Our teachers, who should be helping us develop awareness and skills in interaction and communication, themselves suffer from the same problem. The most they ever do about our talking is to tell us to stop it—while they go on and on and on.

Sometimes it seems that values and expectations are so different from generation to generation that it really is impossible to establish a basis for shared values and understandings. But most of the investigations reveal no great differences. Teenagers are generally very much like their parents in outlook and approach to life. And anyone who suggests that the real gap between the young and the old is an irreconcilable difference in their view of change and their ability to adapt to it are misled by their prejudice. Every 75-year-old living today has adapted to automobiles, electric lights, airplanes, and walks on the moon. And I know many 20-

year-olds who are horrified at the thought of a white woman marrying a black man.

The other day I heard a 70-year-old father arguing with his 50-year-old daughter about her daughter—his granddaughter. It seems that the girl had decided to move from the college dormitory into what she called a community. There, with twelve other young people, she would share the expenses and the chores of living. They would raise their own vegetables, and even help rear two infants of one of the couples.

The woman was distraught, plagued as she was by visions of orgies and decadence that she associated with "communes." The old man was trying to reassure her, urging her to go and see for herself that the lovely child they had both had a hand in educating would not disappoint them. His rationality finally did penetrate her anxiety, and she remembered that the three generations shared the same values.

Given the difficulties of communication that we all have with each other, why are we so particularly susceptible to ambivalence in our relationships with old people? The groundwork for our ambivalence is laid in the precepts of our philosophy: Honor thy father and mother; Forsake all others and follow me; You must show respect for older people—old people. We are prepared for ambivalence also because we live with the fear and threat of death: You'll be sorry when it's too late.

Thus, while the everyday situations in which we find ourselves generate feelings of anger as well as love, annoyance and frustration as well as compassion, we are constrained to express only love and compassion, and to keep what we label "negative" emotions hidden. If we are forever admonished to love our parents, while we lack the skill we need to talk to each other, listen to each other, learn to know each other, we are doomed to veer from love to anger, tenderness to hostility, caring to confusion and frustration in our relationships. But the worldwide movement toward candor and honesty, although it sometimes seems to cause even more difficulties between younger and older people, will eventually help us to deal more effectively with conflicting emotions.

Margaret Mead proposes that the rebellion of young people against the ritual forms for relating to parents and other adults has set us on the road to developing a new kind of relationship between the generations [12]:

> We are moving away from the belief that the mere existence of a biological relationship permits anyone to have an absolute and unqualified claim on the love and concern of another person.
>
> It is reasonable to demand that individuals, whether children or adults, should behave responsibly and humanly toward the people with whom they live or with whom they are associated. I believe this expecta-

tion is slowly coming to replace the idea that one owes a certain kind of behavior to relatives simply because they are relatives. . . .

And I believe parents can learn to treat children, and children can learn to treat parents, as persons.

If our aging and aged parents do indeed become part of our developing humanistic concern for relating to each other openly and with sensitivity, the effect may ultimately be a wider societal move for providing guidelines for later life. This is the significance of dealing here—in a book for nurses—with the problems of ambivalence and communication that adults in general have in their relationship with old people.

Although the nurse functions in a professional milieu, and interacts with old people in a therapeutic relationship, he is still a son, he was once a child, he has dealt—or not dealt—with his own ambivalence toward parents and grandparents, he has experienced the effects of his parents' feelings toward their parents. It is not realistic to expect that he can treat an old person as if all of this did not exist. The chances are that every old person he encounters triggers some memory, some trace of feeling from his personal life. Exhortations to maintain a "professional" stance do not neutralize what he is as a person.

Ambivalence and Social Decision Making

Sharon R. Curtin [13] talks about adult preoccupation with "What To Do with the Old Folks." I think there is a kind of desperation in the preoccupation that comes from the growing awareness that our society provides us with so few guidelines for aging or interacting with the aged. If the pattern and precedents were clear and our education *real*, the anxiety and desperation might be relieved.

For example, as small children we would be respected by our parents (because they were respected by *their* parents and were educated to independence and spontaneity). We would no longer hear: "As long as you live in my house, you'll do as *I* say!" Instead, children would feel comfortable expressing frustration and anger. They would feel free to assert themselves and learn early to assume responsibility for their own decisions. Above all, they would learn to *like* their parents and enjoy their friendship. (Is it so unlikely that people who live together for twenty years, helping each other grow, sharing pleasure and pain, can become fast friends? It requires only a new view of the parent-child relationship, an abandonment of every vestige of the archaic notion that the child *belongs* to his parents.)

The discomfort we experience when, as children, our parents appear in our school or on our ballfields, and the dis-ease when they appear in our homes when we are grown, would disappear.

Although there would probably be parents and children who never become friends, this need not mean that those parents would be abandoned in old age to nursing homes and retirement communities. The age-integrated society that develops out of truly loving child rearing would provide many younger people who would see to it that their old friends were not forgotten. And young people would no longer say to a Margaret Mead, "You belong to us," [14] implying in four words the enormous gap between them and all the other older people.

"Where did I sleep last night?" asked the old man of his son.

"Right here, Dad."

"Where do I go from here?"

"You don't go anywhere. We live here now. We have a two-year lease on the apartment."

"Don't laugh at your old father when he can't remember."

The son couldn't tell if the old man were joking or as serious as his expression—unsmiling, almost glum.

"If you laugh at an old man, you'll be punished. You'll get old yourself."

And the old man laughed.

The development of separate buildings and separate communities for housing old people seems to be part of the nationwide desperation to alleviate the guilt that accompanies ambivalence. Although studies reveal that people who have moved to retirement communities are generally not displeased with their situation, it seems to me that the expressions of acceptance are largely reactive: Since you don't want me to live among you, I prefer to live apart from you. This is a defense mechanism identified by psychologists as the sweet lemon response.

Something of this is revealed in the observations of Bultena and Wood [15]:

> Although only a small proportion of the national aged population is now living in retirement communities, we have found no evidence in our study that these places have a detrimental effect on morale, satisfaction with retirement, or level of social interaction; quite the contrary. . . .
>
> It has been claimed that retirement communities are only an escape from a larger system which excludes older persons from the mainstream of social activity and the central functions of the society. Perhaps this is true. If so, the vehicle that provides escape should not be condemned, but rather the general societal patterns which make such escape desirable today for many older persons.

However, I must say that I *do* "condemn the vehicle." The vehicle helps bolster and perpetuate the system. It helps to keep people from fighting the system.

Those who live in retirement communities are generally better off and better educated than the general aged population. They are well equipped to resist the violation of their dignity by the young and the middle-aged. If they leave and wrap themselves in a soft cocoon of pleasant, aimless living, they deprive the rest of the population of what they know.

In addition, if those who are segregated indeed are *not* aware they are, in effect, on the scrap heap, then the vehicle is to be condemned for keeping them ignorant. In any event, the consequence is a perpetuation of prejudice and discrimination that flourishes when groups are kept separate from each other.

Let us look more closely at this decision we apparently have made to build a segregated world for old people. At every step it reveals clearly that it arises out of the unresolved conflicts in our attitudes toward aging and old age.

In discussing mental health problems of the aged, it has become almost axiomatic that institutionalization as we have seen it in operation is generally harmful. However, "the philosophy of custodialism is so entrenched that benevolent gerontological planners talk about the need to provide custodial care as part of any new comprehensive care system." [16]

Kahn goes on to say that "the negative consequences of mental dysfunction can be minimized by exposing old persons to more demanding and stimulating environments, in contrast to the isolation and dependency effects of the custodial institution. There will be less infantilization and greater opportunities for the old person to maintain control of his own situation." Yet in planning, far greater emphasis—and money—seems to go into ideas for separate housing and institutions than into maintaining people in the environments they chose for themselves originally.

"Ironically, one could question the wisdom of concentrating old people in specific housing. Sweden, for example, has been giving up high-rise enclaves for its older citizens. Rather than a housing program for older citizens, it might be more desirable socially to provide rent supplements or, ultimately, appropriate income maintenance so that the elderly could live anywhere throughout the city. . . . One of the greatest losses of old age is that of choice." [17]

In our whole approach to retirement, we seem to victimize the aged with an ambivalence that transcends individual confusion and is revealed as part of our national dilemma. The work ethic which undergirds our productivity is set in startling contrast to insistence that there is something inherently "natural" about people stopping all work at some arbitrarily designated age. What can we be feeling about people of a certain age when we subject them to the agonies of reconciling a work ethic on which they have been reared with enforced idleness!

"Retirement as it is known today was relatively uncommon in 1900 and the difference between life expectancy and work life expectancy was a scant 3 years." [18] There is a world of difference between spending three years in a "Home" or a retirement community, in a well-earned rest from a life of labor, and the fifteen or twenty years of resting that the contemporary adult faces. So much resting is just too much for the healthy survival of a human being! As Maggie Kuhn says, "But how long can you rest? Resting is deadly." [19]

But there is more to the deadliness than just resting. That part of the ambivalence that is hostility and rejection may be what results in a standard of operation in the institutions—perhaps even in the "senior citizen" housing—that often causes incredible suffering. On a recent television show about nursing homes, an aide in one of them admits in an interview, "I wouldn't have my mother or dad here. . . . I've worked with the girls here, and I know how they work." The examples of "how they work" find their way into almost every publication dealing with aging.

Aides and nurses usually stand while they feed people who may be unable to feed themselves or may simply need more time than others are willing to let them have to feed themselves. There are two practices here that are destructive of dignity: The person who is being fed by someone who is standing cannot help but feel that he is imposing on the time of the feeder, that his eating is just a necessary function rather than a process for enjoyment. It is human beings who make of eating a satisfying social occasion; it is animals who take in food to survive. The old person who is deprived of the social aspects of mealtime is made to feel that much less a person.

In talking to the patients and about them, the attitude of aides and nurses is too often the attitude that adults reveal toward children: they patronize and scold. Symbolic of the adult-child relationship is the form of address: without a by-your-leave, people of 20 call octogenarians by their first names—a nice democratization if the old people were really treated as equals instead of only equally senile.

"Now, finish your oatmeal, Jenny, or you won't be able to go into the sun room with the others."

"Sam, you're being bad, again. You know you make us all unhappy when you're bad."

"Don't you want to look nice when your daughter comes to see you? Let me tie your hair back so it looks right. I don't know why you never let me fix your hair right." (Because, lady, she's always worn her hair quite another way, and she prefers to continue to do so!)

It is not surprising that at least some of the patients tell interviewers that the nurses are *mean*. How many others are afraid to say what they think?

And how many can never again say what they think? Like the patient who may have heard one nurse say to another as they stood at the foot of his bed: "Why don't they let us pull the tube out of his leg and let him die?"

"In a speech to the U.S. House of Representatives on August 3, 1970, Congressman David Pryor of Arkansas reported that we have turned over the sickest, most helpless, and most vulnerable patient group in the medical care system to the most loosely controlled and least responsible faction of that system." [20]

If, in a society, the consequences of ambivalence are lack of communication and hostility, segregation and deprivation, we cannot—as professionals and as individuals, cease in our self-examination and self-evaluation. Above all, we must view with a healthy skepticism the belief that, because we *say* we care about the aged, and we teach the humanistic treatment of the aged, we all practice what we profess.

Notes

1. Donald Kent, "Aging: Fact and Fantasy," *The Gerontologist,* Vol. 5, No. 2, June, 1965, pp. 51–56, 111.

2. Bernice L. Neugarten, "Social Implications of a Prolonged Life-Span," *The Gerontologist,* Vol. 12, No. 3, Part IV, Winter, 1972, pp. 323–440.

3. Margaret Mead, *Blackberry Winter—My Earlier Years,* William Morrow & Co., Inc., New York, 1972, p. 45.

4. Ibid., p. 53.

5. Margaret Mead, "Celebrating the Bicentennial—Family Style," *Redbook,* April, 1975, pp. 31, 33, 37.

6. Margaret Mead and Ken Heyman, *Family,* Macmillan Publishing Co., Inc., New York, 1965, p. 84.

7. Mead, "Celebrating the Bicentennial," op. cit.

8. Mead and Hyman, op. cit., p. 84.

9. Mead, *Blackberry Winter,* op. cit., p. 56.

10. Robert N. Butler, "Age-ism: Another Form of Bigotry," *The Gerontologist,* Vol. 9, Part I, 1969, pp. 243–246.

11. Bartram B. Moss, with Kent Fraser, *Caring for the Aged,* Doubleday & Company, Inc., New York, 1966, p. 102.

12. Margaret Mead, "Margaret Mead Answers," *Redbook,* July 1974, pp. 33–34, 37.

13. Sharon R. Curtin, *Nobody Ever Died of Old Age,* Little, Brown and Company, Boston, 1972.

14. Margaret Mead, *Culture and Commitment,* Natural History Press, Garden City, N.Y., 1970, p. 95.

15. Gordon L. Bultena and Vivian Wood, "The American Retirement Community: Bane or Blessing?" *Journal of Gerontology,* Vol. 24, No. 2, April, 1969, pp. 209–217.

16. Robert L. Kahn, "The Mental Health System and the Future Aged," *The Gerontologist,* February, 1975 (Supplement), pp. 24–31.

17. Butler, op. cit.

18. U.S. Department of Labor, Manpower Report No. 8, *The Length of Working Life for Males, 1900–1960,* Washington, D.C., July, 1963, pp. 7–8.

19. Bill Mandel, "What Makes Maggie Kuhn Gallop—at 69?" *The Philadelphia Inquirer,* April 27, 1975, p.1I, 8I.

20. Bert Kruger Smith, *Aging in America,* Beacon Press, Boston, 1973, pp. 68–69.

2

*exercises in awareness
and skill development*

*the functioning
of ambivalence*

A Note on Role Confusion

Where it comes to defining the role of the nurse in sociological terms, there is widespread consensus on most aspects of the role. It is easy to identify most behaviors of nurses and get agreement from professionals and lay people alike as to the appropriateness of the functions. Except when we come to some of the new extensions of the nursing function, like midwifery, there is very little role conflict in the nursing profession.

If this is true, what prevents a particular nurse from fulfilling the role expectations of her profession? The general societal ambivalence toward aging, old age, and old people intervene when the nurse comes into contact with a patient who is old, and her confusion can cause inappropriate role behavior.

For example, if our society is not sure whether old people are all experienced, wise, and capable of controlling their own lives, or childish, incompetent, and dependent, the nurse may find herself seesawing between helping the patient maintain his independence and forcing him to submit completely to her will. If the role expectations of nursing demand that the nurse foster independence, this nurse's controlling behavior is inappropriate. If the role expectations of nursing demand that the patient be treated in terms of his needs, this nurse's obvious confusion about the patient's needs has led to inappropriate behavior.

From a somewhat different point of view, the nurse who has not resolved his personal conflicts about his relationship with the old people in his life, or his anxiety about his own aging, may also demonstrate some role confusion. For example, his pity for a man just because he is old, and his discomfort in that same man's presence because age frightens him, can cause him one moment to be too nurturing, too protective, and the next moment to avoid the patient and so deprive him of needed care. Or, a father neglected in old age may cause such guilt that a patient who is old becomes sometimes the surrogate father and other times the target of hostility.

In this chapter, we are interested in helping nurses identify a variety of behaviors that arise out of ambivalence toward old people, helping them to feel something of the effects of such behaviors, and then to obtain information about what is reflected in their own behaviors. The hope is that raised consciousness, together with development of empathy, will prepare the way for whatever changes nurses desire to make in their own professional functioning.

Identifying Behaviors

Following are a number of case studies that illustrate the behaviors resulting from ambivalence. After each case is an analysis pointing out the triggers that release first one behavior and then another—contradictory—behavior in the ambivalent person.

Read the first case and its analysis, then try to analyze each of the other cases before you read the text version. The following questions may provide some help in identifying the ambivalent behaviors and their triggers:

1. What do you know of the nurse's (doctor's, therapist's) attitude toward people generally?
2. Can you identify specific behaviors that reveal this attitude? (The *expression* of ideas, beliefs, etc., may be considered to be a behavior.)
3. What do you know of the nurse's (doctor's) feeling about herself?
4. Can you identify specific behaviors that reveal this attitude?
5. What is the nurse's (doctor's, therapist's) attitude toward the other person in the case study?
6. Is there evidence that the attitude is not consistent?
7. Can you identify specific behaviors that reveal the contradictory aspects of this attitude?

Case No. 1

Mrs. Rason is a nurse recognized by her colleagues and by the patients she treats as extremely knowledgeable and competent. She never "cuts corners" in the care of patients but follows orders and takes initiatives so that she provides a very high level of nursing care.

Miss Sinavan is 68 years old. She has been admitted to the hospital for a series of diagnostic tests to determine the cause of persistent and debilitating dizziness. Although she seems perfectly all right for hours at a time, she may suddenly become dizzy and fall if there are no supports nearby. She has already bruised herself severely in several places, and both she and her doctor are afraid that she may hurt herself badly in one of these falls.

As usual, Mrs. Rason is doing everything possible to make Miss Sinavan comfortable. Not only does she follow the medical orders meticulously, but she bathes her patient every day, sees to it that the bed linens are smooth and comfortable. When Miss Sinavan is in bed, Mrs. Rason comes in regularly to encourage her to change her position; when she walks, the nurse makes sure that someone is close to her at all times. Through all her ministrations, Mrs. Rason is smiling, calm, receptive to what the patient says and is in all ways an exemplary professional.

The other day, had anyone been observing, he might have recorded the following conversation between Mrs. Rason and her patient:

MRS. RASON: Good morning, Josephine! Isn't it a lovely morning?

MISS SINAVAN: It is! It's a shame to be indoors on a day like this.

MRS. RASON: Oh, I don't know. I like working—especially with such nice people—like you.

MISS SINAVAN: You're a wonderful nurse. Everyone says so.

MRS. RASON: *(relaxing against the foot of the bed)* I hear you're pretty good at *your* profession. Some of your visitors have been talking.

MISS SINAVAN: It's easier for me. I don't have to deal with people who are sick and unhappy.

MRS. RASON: It's working with people and knowing you can help them. I guess that's what keeps us both going.

MISS SINAVAN: *(smiling)* I know you keep a lot of people going.

MRS. RASON: Well, well! Let's end the mutual admiration meeting and get on with the business at hand. It's time for your bath. Let me help you off with your gown.

MISS SINAVAN: I think I can get it off by myself.

MRS. RASON: *(removing the gown)* There you are! Now, wasn't that easy? Come along, now. We'll get you into the tub and washed.

MISS SINAVAN: Please. Can't you just stay nearby in case I get dizzy? But let me bathe myself? I really don't feel like an invalid.

MRS. RASON: Now, now, let's not be grumpy. I have a lot to do this morning.

MISS SINAVAN: I can bathe myself!

MRS. RASON: I'm surprised at you, Josephine! I thought you were one of the cooperative patients!

MISS SINAVAN: I don't see why. . . .

MRS. RASON: I don't have time for this nonsense! You're taking time from my other patients! Now, do you do as I ask, or do we forget the whole thing?!

MISS SINAVAN: *(dejected)* I'm sorry! I didn't mean to interfere with the routine.

MRS. RASON: Oh, please. I didn't mean to fly off the handle like that.

Sometimes I give the impression I'm really angry. But I'm not. *(smiling)* Come along. I'll bathe you now and make you feel better.

Analysis of Case No. 1

Mrs. Rason obviously cares about her patients. She enjoys her work and appreciates the opportunity to interact with the people with whom she comes into contact. She takes the time for casual pleasantries and responds in kind to friendly overtures. (The fact that she is competent in the technical aspects of her profession contributes to her sense of confidence and makes her able to relax occasionally, secure in the knowledge that everyone recognizes that the job is getting done in the best possible way.)

Since her conception of her professional self seems realistic and healthy, the sudden anger at Miss Sinavan's resistance to her wishes does not seem to come from self-doubt. She does not seem to be afraid that if she doesn't keep absolute control over everybody and everything, she will be unable to function. Yet she responds with sudden anger at Miss Sinavan's insistence that she not be treated as if she were a helpless invalid.

Is it possible that Miss Sinavan's self-assertion simply does not fit in with Mrs. Rason's expectation of appropriate behavior? Is it that she believes that all patients should be passive and dependent, or does she feel that way only about older patients? Is her picture of older people one of retirement, helplessness, inability to function independently? Does she get upset when an old person doesn't conform to that picture?

Perhaps her confidence in her knowledge and skill *is* threatened when the behavior of an individual seems to demonstrate that her own knowledge is not absolute. Mrs. Rason really likes Miss Sinavan, and accepts her. The older woman's obvious independence triggers the nurse's behaviors of dislike and rejection. Compliance with her wishes immediately results in the liking, accepting behaviors again.

Case No. 2

The old man propped up in the hospital bed nods and smiles at the young nurse. His trembling hands take one of hers, holding and patting it gently as he speaks.

"My dear child," he says. "Let an old man advise you. Don't let these things bother you."

The nurse smiles tremulously. "I can't help it," she says. "That man upsets me so! Nothing I do pleases him."

"Well, he's a big doctor. Big doctors have a lot on their minds. He doesn't mean to hurt you."

"Oh, Mr. Lavene, I'm so unhappy!" She is almost in tears, almost— but not quite—asking to be embraced and comforted.

The tremor that was only in the patient's hands is now reflected in the shaking of his head. He is very tired. But the nurse's awareness is turned inward. She details the outrages heaped on her by the resident on the floor.

"He's always criticizing what I do! I'm beginning to feel that I don't know anything about nursing! And he expects me to be everywhere at once! If I'm not right there when he wants something, he yells at me as if I were off somewhere having a good time. I can't be in two places at one time!"

The old man's eyes close—then open with great effort. The second or third time this happens, the nurse suddenly seems to become aware of her patient's fatigue. She says nothing more—just pats his hand, lowers the bed, and closes the window blind. She seems a little downcast as she quietly closes the door of the room behind her.

Before you read what follows, go back to the questions at the beginning of the exercise, and use them as guidelines for doing your own analysis of this case. Then you might compare your analysis with the one that follows.

Do this with each of the cases in this chapter.

Analysis of Case No. 2

There is no evidence here that the nurse is suffering more than the usual kind of frustration resulting from human interaction. In one situation a teacher is unfair, in another, an employer is inconsiderate, in another a parent does not understand. These are the daily problems with which all of us must cope.

The nurse in this situation has found a way to cope with a difficult colleague: she finds a "father" and cries on his shoulder. For a while, she is again a child finding sympathy and comfort in the arms of an uncritical, omniscient parent. So absorbed is she in her role playing that she misinterprets the polite response of a stranger, and forgets for a while that the old man is her patient, that *he* is in need of *her* nurturing.

Is this just a momentary lapse on the part of the nurse, a brief response to overwhelming pressure, quickly extinguished and never to be repeated? Or is it evidence of a certain expectation in her relationships with old people? Does she see in every older person a stereotype of the wise and comforting parent who will, upon demand, subordinate his own needs and concerns to hers? Is she so committed to this image that, when she is troubled, *she* subordinates the nurse-patient relationship to the parent-child one?

Obviously, she recalls herself to the reality; the symptoms of illness pierce her preoccupation and she springs back into the professional role. However, she is left with a feeling of sadness—a sense of loss at losing a parent.

Case No. 3

The physician was very kind as he sat and talked with the old man's daughter. He sympathized with her sorrow; he knew how much she loved her father.

"There is really no other way," he told her sadly. "He'll be like a child."

"Do you mean there's no chance he will ever be better?"

"Well, if he improves, he improves. There's nothing we can treat, if that's what you mean. The chances are, however, that he has recouped as much of his mental ability as he ever will. After all, he's 85 years old!"

"But he's always been in good health. There's never been anything seriously wrong with him."

"Believe me. A nursing home is the best place for him. If, by some wild chance, he does improve, you can always take him home."

"No," she said firmly. Almost, he could detect hostility in her stiff back and unsmiling face. "I wouldn't do that to anyone. Certainly not to my own father."

A fleeting frown of annoyance passed across his face. But he was all kindness and concern again. "Nursing homes were designed specifically for this kind of situation. He'll be cared for; and you can visit him regularly."

"But look how much better he is since it happened. After the seizure he couldn't even speak or understand what was said to him. Now he speaks perfectly well!"

"That's true. But he's had extensive brain damage and he'll never be what he was."

"I think that if he's at home with people he loves, he may improve even more."

"He'll get good care in the Home."

"But he'll just sit around there, with people he doesn't know. Isn't it better for him to have the normal kind of company, and things to do around the house? Doesn't just taking him away from his family have a bad effect?"

The physician seemed to pull back physically. Again the annoyance flashed on his face and disappeared.

"It's true that most nursing homes don't offer the stimulation and interest that keep old people from deteriorating further, but how much difference can it make to him? He'll be comfortable, his meals will be served to him. He'll be fine," he finished heartily.

"I really don't understand you, Doctor," the young woman looked searchingly into his face. "You admit that being in a Home may make him worse, but you're telling me not to take him home to live with me. I just don't understand."

"Well, I don't know what your social position is, but. . . ."

He stopped short at the look of incredulity he saw.

"I mean, as long as you can afford to get him cared for. . . ."

But the young woman was on her feet, signaling an end to the interview.

"If you'll just let me know when he's ready to be discharged, Doctor. I won't take up any more of your time."

The doctor shrugged his shoulders as he watched her leave. He seemed to be thinking that he had done his best to give sensible advice and that it was no concern of his if the fool woman wouldn't take that advice. But he also seemed to be shrugging off the vague feeling of unease that her reaction had left in him.

Analysis of Case No. 3

Here the ambivalence to be inferred from the physician's behavior is not so much precipitated by the responses of the patient's daughter. It seems, rather, to manifest itself as he, himself, tries to maintain some consistency in his position vis-à-vis institutionalization of old people.

His immediate recommendation is that the patient be institutionalized, but he finds it difficult to justify that recommendation on medical grounds. His point of view apparently is based in a values orientation— and his values are coming into conflict with his medical knowledge. On the one hand, he has evidence that long-term institutionalization generally has a debilitating effect on old people, who suffer there from sensory deprivation with its attendant loss of interest, initiative, and even motivation to move. Although it is difficult always to document the psychological and physical deterioration without controlled comparative data, there are logical inferences to be made: it is quite possible that at least some deterioration is preventable in a stimulating atmosphere.

This is aside from consideration of the salutary effects of living with loved ones, as opposed to living with strangers—and having an opportunity to interact in personal and social functions with people of all ages.

We can assume that a competent, well-trained physician has had, in his background, some exposure to this kind of information and the inferences to be drawn from it. On the other hand, he reveals the cultural reluctance to permit an old person to share his life, the cultural assumption that an old person will probably never be "better," the cultural belief that an old person has lived as long as he should. These cultural values become the basis of his professional advice.

The discomfort he seems to feel, the startled annoyance he experiences when his advice is challenged, are the result of conflict between his knowledge and his feelings.

Case No. 4

Ms. Singer is a teacher of nurses in the baccalaureate program of a large university. One of the sections in her course on Care of the Chronically Ill is devoted to geriatrics. In it, she brings to the students the latest research findings on aging, examines with them the current practices in the care of the aged and, in conjunction with the university hospital, provides an opportunity for them to have some experience nursing old people. She often marvels at the image of objectivity and sagacity she presents in class, when at the same time she is so torn with ambivalent feelings toward her father and self-blame for her behavior.

Here is a record of an incident involving her and her 85-year-old father, who has just come to live with her after suffering a stroke that caused brain damage. He now cannot remember recent events, often does not know where he is, and, if left alone for long periods of time becomes anxious almost to the point of panic.

NURSE: I'm going out for the evening, Dad. Some friends are coming by for me, and we're going to dinner and a show. All right, Dad?

FATHER: Of course it's all right! You do anything you have to do.

NURSE: I'll call you during the evening.

FATHER: Take care of yourself.

NURSE: I will. (*Kisses him good night and opens the door. Hesitates at the door, turns and looks back at him. He is not looking at her. She sighs and leaves, closing the door behind her.)*

At the end of her dinner, and then during each intermission at the show, she dashed to the phone to call him. Each time he was watching television, he was looking at the newspaper, he was fine.

When she got home (fifteen minutes after the curtain rang down—no restaurant, no leisurely after-theater drink) her father was lying on the living room sofa. All the lights were out, but he obviously wasn't asleep.

NURSE: Daddy, are you all right? *(on the edge of panic)*

FATHER: All right.

NURSE: Why are you lying in the dark?

FATHER: I wanted to lie down.

NURSE: You never go to sleep so early. You always watch television. Why aren't you watching?

FATHER: I don't feel well.

NURSE: What's bothering you? Does something hurt you?

FATHER: Yes. Everything.

NURSE: Can you point to where it hurts?

FATHER: I can't exactly tell you.

NURSE: Why don't you get up and get undressed and go to bed? You'll be more comfortable.

Ten minutes later he is sitting up, the room is brightly lit, and he is watching a police story.

NURSE: Would you like something to eat or drink?

FATHER: Yes. I'd like a cup of coffee.

She busies herself making the coffee. There seems to be more rattling of pots and banging of cutlery than usual. Finally, she brings the coffee, putting it down with some emphasis in front of her father.

NURSE: Here's the coffee. Well, aren't you going to drink it?

FATHER: Yes, of course. Thank you, dear.

NURSE: If you wanted coffee, why didn't you make yourself a cup?

FATHER: What?

NURSE: Why do you have to wait until I ask you? You could have had coffee an hour ago!

FATHER: I know. I didn't want it earlier.

NURSE: No—you didn't want it! You just wanted to lie in the dark and feel sorry for yourself!

FATHER: I didn't feel well.

NURSE: You feel perfectly all right now! You recover completely five minutes after I come home! *(her voice has risen almost to a shout)*

FATHER: I just love to see you. *I* feel at home when I see you!

NURSE: *(in a lower-than-normal voice)* Oh, Daddy, I know. *(puts her arms around him)* But I can't be with you all the time.

FATHER: I don't expect you to. I know you have things to do. I love you very much. You're the best daughter a man can have. You couldn't do any more for me than you do.

NURSE: I love you, too, Daddy. You're very good. You take my yelling and irritability and you don't get angry with me.

FATHER: I love you. I understand.

Analysis of Case No. 4

Here is the way Ms. Singer analyzes her own feelings toward her father:

For the first time in my life I am fully aware of the meaning of the word "ambivalence." I know I love my father. I care about his aches and pains. I worry about whether or not he will ever really be himself again. I am overjoyed each time I see some sign that his memory is improving or that his pains are diminishing. But there are times when I resent him, resent the limits in my movement caused by his presence. I resent having to get up each morning and prepare breakfast and lunch, when I'm frantic to get at the pile of work on my desk. I resent not being able to accept a speaking engagement in another state, because I haven't yet figured out how to provide for his care while I'm gone.

On a more profound level, I hate it—and sometimes I think I hate him—because he didn't provide for his own old age. Oh, I don't mean financially. I mean psychologically and—if you like—socially. He shouldn't be living with a daughter—someone who is impatient to get on with her own life, someone to whom any attachment is an encumbrance. He should be living with a wife, someone who is prepared to spend most of her time doing with him and for him. I know it would be healthier for him to be living with a woman, instead of living with a daughter he sometimes perceives as his companion, sharing his life in a way that no daughter wants to.

The biggest problem is that he has no one else to interact with. He suddenly finds himself in a city he never lived in, with no one he knows, no friends or acquaintances. And he has never been what you would call gregarious. Now there is no chance of his making friends. He can sit surrounded by people in the park or the lobby of the apartment house, and never dream of venturing to say a word—or even to make eye contact—with a single person. Even if I speak to people and draw them close, his complete nonparticipation in the conversation discourages them from making any overtures toward him.

The burden of his isolation on me is enormous. This, more than anything else, is forcing me to severely limit my own life, because I feel obliged to go home whenever I don't absolutely have to work. I never was a gadabout before, but now I spend almost all my nonworking time at home with him, because I know how lonely he must be.

And sometimes when I sit and look at him, so quiet, so patient with what must be his agonizing confusion and frustration, I'm overwhelmed with such love and pity that I can hardly stand it.

I think nothing frustrates, infuriates, and makes me cry as much as coming home to find him sitting—or lying wide-awake—in the dark. Nothing is so calculated to make me feel guilty as this picture of quiet, lonely suffering. Once I yelled a lot at him, some confused demand that he "once, just once, ask me if I had a good time, or what I did!" He had an answer to that, of course: he didn't want to interfere; he didn't want to pry into my activities! And I had an answer for that: he just wasn't interested enough in what I did. Didn't care whether or not I had a good time!

Intellectually, I know that ambivalence not infrequently characterizes the relationships between parents and children. Love/hate is often fostered by the loving nurturing and the noncommunication and misunderstandings during the growing-up period. In adulthood the conflicting feelings are reinforced by the discomforts of the present.

It worries me: Am I as accepting of my older patients, as consistent in my behavior as I think I am? Do I interact with them in the ways prescribed in my lectures to the students. Or do my professional relationships reflect my personal one? Is my ambivalence only personal and apparent in my attitude toward my father, or is it a part of my feelings about all old people?

I don't know. . . .

Case No. 5

The inhalation therapist was very gentle with the old woman. He was reluctant to wake her from restful sleep in order to treat her, and he came back several times to see if she had wakened by herself. Finally, he approached her quietly, put his hand on her cheek and called her name softly. She woke smiling, recognized him immediately, and asked if it was time again for her "breathing."

"That's right, Molly," he answered. "You were fast asleep, weren't you. Naughty girl! You should be up and waiting for me!"

Mrs. Abram's smile was a little smaller. "I'm sorry," she answered. "I'm afraid I don't really know your schedule."

"Now, now! Let's not get *too* nosy. Next thing you'll be doing is ducking out when you know I'm coming."

"Why would I do that?" Mrs. Abrams murmured. She was no longer smiling.

"Just the natural desire to play hookey. . . . Isn't that what kids do?"

"Kids?"

"Oh, come along, now. Don't pout. Let me see you smile! I can't do my work unless you smile!"

Mrs. Abrams said nothing, but submitted patiently to the therapy. Later, she heard the therapist talking to someone in the corridor outside her door.

"I just *love* old people, don't you? They're so *cute!*" (*an unintelligible murmur in response*)

"Oh, they're just like small children! I can usually coax them around to cooperate with me."

(*murmur*)

"The point is, they *know* I *love* them. I really do. They can sense that, so we always have a very good relationship.

Analysis of Case No. 5

What is the connection between love and denigration? How can it be so easy to seesaw between honest feelings and expression of affection at one moment and insulting, ego-destroying behaviors the next moment?

Part of it must arise from a misconception of what the old person is really like. The belief, for example, that all old people are like children will justify behavior vis-à-vis the old that can have the effect of humiliating and infuriating them. Take the nurse in the following situation [1]:

INTERVIEWER: You work almost entirely with old people. Do you like this kind of patient population?

NURSE: Well, actually, I majored in peds. I was sure I'd spend my professional life working with children. I really loved it.

INTERVIEWER: Didn't you find it difficult to make the change? From one extreme to the other?

Nurse: Oh, no. There's really no difference. I get along just fine with old people. The psychology is the same—for children and for old people.

Such a nurse will feel perfectly comfortable responding to an old man in the same way as she would respond to a small child: "Eat your spinach or there'll be no TV tonight." To speak to a child in this way is, at least, culturally acceptable, although it is doubtful that this is the best way to help a child to learn what he needs in order to live independently and productively. But to an adult, the approach is an outrage, implying as it does that (1) he cannot rationally utilize factual data (the food is a vital factor in his recovery), (2) that anyone has the right to deprive him of TV without his compliance, and (3) that anyone has the right to force his compliance with a threat. There *must* be contempt for such an image of an adult.

The affection that is felt—and expressed—is the affection for people in general, together with the cultural admonition to love and respect the old, together, too, with one's own memories of and experiences with grandparents and other aged relatives.

The inhalation therapist "really" does feel warmth and love for old people. Perhaps he misses the grandparents he never knew, and feels some deprivation when he recalls the stories his parents told him about *their* parents in the old country. His lack of personal experience with aged relatives has led him, since childhood, to fantasize about "sitting at a grandmother's knee." Or, perhaps he does remember his grandparents, or an aged great-aunt or uncle, and he transfers the love he had for them to the patients he treats. But, though he knew his own relatives as unique individuals, the psychological pressures of our culture may have blurred his perceptions, and, from a distance he sees his relatives as exceptions to the rule that old people are all alike, lovable but inferior.

A nurse in a doctor's office witnessed an incident that demonstrates this almost frightening kind of inconsistency:

> The overdependent, terrified old man who sat next to his wife in the doctor's waiting room was obviously resented to the point of hatred by his wife.
>
> "What are we waiting for?" he asked her for the fifth time since I had been sitting there.
>
> "Just be quiet!" she almost shouted at him. "There are other people here! Stop making a fool of yourself!"
>
> "I'm sorry. Don't be angry."
>
> And again he asked, "What are we waiting for?"
>
> "Do you want me to get up and leave you, right now?"
>
> He looked terribly frightened, and I could read on his face the

anxiety that I am sure he must have expressed to her countless times, "You won't throw me out, will you? You won't send me to a Home?"

The doctor told me later, "I tell her not to take what he says personally. He can't help it—he just can't help it. But she keeps complaining that it's driving her up the wall. I *tell* her he can't help it."

But she must have known this at some level of awareness. Because a minute after her last threat, apparently when she saw the look of fear on his face, she had put her arms around him and rocked with him as she murmured, "It's all right. Don't worry. We'll go home soon and have dinner. I have your favorite dinner tonight."

And she held him until he no longer seemed afraid.

Developing Empathy

Sometimes, just reading about people who demonstrate certain behaviors and analyzing what we read does not ensure that we will feel the distress of those who are in conflict or are being victimized by another's conflict. Since we cannot really take over another person's body and feelings, we must compromise by trying to get a little closer to knowing what it is to be someone else. Simulating a situation and taking the role of another person often provides us with insights that we have been unable to get in other ways.

It is important to remember that one of the advantages of role playing is that it is much safer than living through the real situation. Destructive behavior is only simulated, and new behaviors can be "tried on," tested out, and kept or discarded as we note their effects. To maintain this level of safety, observers must be cautioned to do nothing to interfere with the role playing—from coaching the players to blaming them for not doing the "right" thing. The function of the observers is to pick up on aspects of the observed relationships for purposes of identifying behaviors—their causes and effects—and thinking up behaviors that might make the relationship more productive and satisfying.

1. Using each case in the preceding section, have someone take each role in the situation and play out the scene, extending it in any way that seems appropriate. Through it all, the ambivalent role player should try to demonstrate her ambivalence, veering from one feeling to another as the other role player's behavior provides the stimulus that releases the ambivalence.
2. The rest of the group is to write down its observations: the behaviors revealing ambivalence and the effects of those behaviors.
3. After playing the scene, let the role players say how they felt. Then let the same role players replay the scene, this time trying to change the nature of the interaction so that the evidence of ambivalence does not emerge.

4. Again, let the role players say how they felt.
5. Let the observers share their observations.
6. Both the observers and the role players discuss the effects on the characters of the change. Are the results constructive or destructive? Is the relationship improved or does it deteriorate?
7. Is there still another way to play out the scene? Perhaps some of the observers would like to try an alternative way.
8. After each role-playing attempt, let the role players say how they feel.

Gathering Data to Control Ambivalence

1. Observation and Feedback

The most direct and productive way to identify our own ambivalent behaviors is to ask a knowledgeable, and nonthreatening, colleague to observe us in an interactive situation. Although we may learn quickly to recognize and analyze ambivalent behavior in hypothetical cases, it is easy to fall into the practice of rationalizing our own behavior: finding acceptable reasons why the way we behave is the only way that is logical or possible.

To reduce the level of threat in an observation, it might be useful to pair up with someone and take turns observing each other and giving each other feedback on observations. The shared vulnerability may keep caustic criticism and denigrating evaluations to a minimum, and encourage the nonevaluative identification of behaviors for the information and use of the person observed.

A colleague observing us may raise in our minds questions about certain aspects of our interaction. How we answer those questions, and whether or not we modify our behavior, is of course, in the final analysis, up to each of us.

The checklist of behaviors that follows may help in the observation process. However, do not hesitate to note other behaviors that seem to reveal ambivalence but are not listed here. The plan for observation should provide for an extended period of time with all the people (patients, colleagues, relatives, and friends of patients) who are identified as old. Since ambivalence may not become apparent during every interaction, if the observer is to get all the possible data, he must accompany the person observed on all professional duties during the course of a working week, or even two weeks.

It should not be very difficult to arrange this for students, assigning them in pairs for the required period of time. For in-service observation, it may be necessary to pair up with someone in the same department and on the same working shift, arranging in advance for the person to be present only during those times when an old person is being interacted with.

Some of the spontaneity of interaction may be sacrificed in this sporadic observation, but it can be revived if the observation time is extended to several weeks so that the two professionals become accustomed to the pattern of planning ahead for observation, and having an observer present for only part of the working time.

Checklist of Ambivalent Behaviors

Check
here

1. Says patient should learn, but prevents learning by anger.
   Further description of situation: _____

2. Says patient should learn, but prevents learning by denigration.
   Further description of situation: _____

3. Says patient should learn, but prevents learning by impatience.
   Further description of situation: _____

4. Says patient should learn, but provides no opportunity.
   Further description of situation: _____

5. Expresses affection but violates dignity.
   Further description of situation: _____

6. Expresses affection but assumes incompetence.
   Further description of situation: _____

7. Expresses affection but reveals hostility.
   Further description of situation: _____

8. Expresses affection but circumscribes relationship.
   Further description of situation: _____

9. Steps out of professional role and assumes role of offspring.
   Further description of situation: _____

10. Steps out of professional role and assumes role of intimate friend.
    Further description of situation: _____

11. Steps out of professional role and assumes role of close relative.
    Further description of situation: _____

12. Steps out of professional role and assumes role of advisor on
ancillary matters.
Further description of situation: _____

13. Expresses views that are intellectually and emotionally conflicting.
Further description of situation: _____

14. Encourages independence and prevents independence.
Further description of situation: _____

Some Notes on the Checklist Items

1–3. The anger of the teacher can be used in such a way that learning is directly inhibited. For example, if the patient insists on doing
something for himself, the nurse may say, "All right. Go ahead! Why
don't you do it, then? If you think you can, go ahead!" If the patient
asks for help on some facet of the process, the nurse may say, "Don't ask
me! You're the one who didn't want any help! See, you *can't* do it alone!
Next time, maybe you'll listen to me!"

The "reason" for the anger often seems obvious: the individual expects too much of others, the individual imposes on others unnecessarily,
the individual refuses to cooperate, the individual interferes with the
routine. The "teacher" may not be aware of the real reason, which is
probably his need to keep the patient dependent on him. Or he may
nurture the expectation that "such" people are inevitably unable to maintain independence; by his behavior he becomes the agent for fulfilling his
own expectation.

4. We all know the people who keep grumbling about what other
people do not know. Often, it is merely an effort to call attention to how
much the grumbler knows—how much more he knows than those others.
Obviously, if he gave the others an opportunity to learn, they would no
longer suffer by comparison to him.

It may be, however, that the nurse has just lost sight of his teaching
function. He forgets that there are many skills that he takes for granted
in himself that other people need instruction in and time to learn.

Also, the urgent press of duties often forces professionals to concentrate on getting the job done. Not infrequently, the job gets done at the
expense of the people for whose benefit the job is *supposed* to be. The
thirty children in a classroom who are taught as if they were all the
same, and nurses' aides who bathe old people on an assembly line are

assuming that, even if they were given creative opportunity and time, neither the "slow" children nor the old people will learn.

5, 6. Dressing old women up with bows in their hair or ignoring the habits of modesty old men have maintained in a lifetime are both assaults on dignity and the sense of self-worth. Old people are not "cute," nor are they inured to the sensitivities they developed in their youth. Assaults on the self-worth of others is not compatible with protestations of affection.

7. Hostility may be felt by the professional for any one of countless reasons, from unresolved childhood conflicts to merely hating the work. Because it is impossible to avoid or ignore the patient, he may become the fortuitous target of the spillover of hostile feelings. Here, again, *after the fact,* conditions and circumstances are identified as justifying the hostility, so that the conscience of the professional may be relieved of guilt.

Not only do we, as professionals, need to develop skills in identifying our own defense mechanisms, but we should provide opportunity for potential victims to speak out when they are unjustly attacked. However, like children in the classroom, the patient often feels powerless to assert himself, fearful of the consequences of such assertion. The teacher, or the nurse, has a significant role to play in helping to free his pupils—his patients—from such fears.

8–12. Although we must recognize that we cannot establish close personal relationships with all our patients, clients, and students, professionals in all fields need to reexamine the position at which they draw the line that separates their professional from their personal relationships.

There appears to be some confusion about what a "professional" relationship requires. Often, this seems to mean that communication with the patient is stripped down to the essentials of direction giving, sprinkled with a few noncommittal comments on the weather. When some people, in a violent reaction against this minimal level of communication, attempt to humanize their interaction with patients, they permit a blurring of the professional role until it is no longer recognizable. The therapeutic function jockeys for precedence with the personal needs of the professional. Unjustifiable demands are unconsciously made on the patient, not least among which are the demands that he permit the therapist to displace the significant people in his life.

Thus, the nurse not only expects the patient to share with him the intimate details of his personal life, but he—as a close friend would—offers the details of his own life to the patient. Thus, too, the nurse not only invites the patient's expression of concern about her children, but—as a sister does—gives unsolicited advice about management, punishment, and relationship with the divorced father.

Although the roles of friend, confidante, and advisor do not always necessarily conflict with the role of therapist, it is when the therapist assumes these roles, not as a response to the needs of the patient, but in response to his own needs, that the conflict becomes apparent.

13,14. The American conflict between the intellectual and the emotional was long ago recognized by Gunnar Myrdal and graphically identified as the *American Dilemma*. On the one hand, we believe in the essential equality of all human beings and we have scientific data that undergird this belief; on the other hand, we treat some people, interact with them, as if they were another, inferior, species. Myrdal, of course, dealt with the white dilemma concerning black people. But the analogy for the attitude of younger people toward the old is not so farfetched.

Nurses and other professionals have access to the newest knowledge about aging and people who are old. Yet they often respond to old people in terms of archaic attitudes learned in childhood and reinforced by the media, and by the prevailing cultural attitudes.

The ambivalence becomes apparent when, in discussions with colleagues, the professional may, for example, assert strongly that an old person may or may not be self-assertive, independent, capable, and desirous of managing his own life. The nurse may be intellectually aware of the fact that a random sample of people over 65 or 75 will reveal the whole range of independence. But, in practice, it will become apparent that he operates on another level, treating all old people as if they are incapable of assuming control over even the smallest decision.

A more extreme form of this kind of ambivalence (which more obviously assumes the form of traditional prejudice) is seen in the individual who believes the stereotypes about old people but is receptive to the palpable evidence that a *particular* old person does not fit the stereotype. Such an individual is willing to admit that this violation of the stereotype is merely an "exception." So he will, for example, permit the "exception" to maintain his independence, while every other old person he encounters must begin from scratch to prove that he is also an "exception" to the stereotype.

2. Self-Observation

An alternative to working with a colleague to identify ambivalent behavior is, of course, to check one's own behavior. This may present some difficulties because we have a tendency to select out of what we do and what we see those factors that do not fit our preconceptions, our desires, our anxieties. Thus, if we say or do something that is not consistent with our picture of ourselves, we may actively "forget" that we have said or done it. Or we may think we observed some behavior in the patient that justifiably evoked our own response. Since we all have a tendency to perceive selectively in this way, the margin for error in self-observation is bound to be greater without at least one other person to corroborate the accuracy of the observation.

However, the advantages of self-observation are also to be considered. There is usually less anxiety and feeling of threat if we are not exposing ourselves to the possibility of another person's evaluation (although it should be borne in mind that there are always other people around observing our behavior. They may not always let us know what they think of it, but their judgments inevitably influence their behavior in relating to us.)

Self-observation permits continuous observation for a period of time, during which major focus is on ourselves. Even with a peer assigned to the same area, that person will probably be performing other professional duties and may miss some of the things you do and say.

Self-observation leaves one freer to develop his own priorities and patterns for changing. The commitment to yourself to change, and the knowledge of how you can best succeed in making the changes you want are unfettered by the need to "prove" something to someone else or the pressure to make the changes someone else sees as most important. This is, I think, consistent with any definition of professionalism: the true professional is forever becoming—learning, developing skills, sharpening sensitivities. And he does this out of his commitment to the work he has undertaken.

One procedural note on using the checklist of ambivalent behaviors: It is advisable to check the item and describe the situation as soon as possible after it happens, or the incident—or details of it—may be forgotten.

Without the check on subjectivity that another observer offers, it might even be better to forego the use of the checklist of ambivalent behaviors and, instead, describe in detail each ten- or fifteen-minute interaction with a person who is old. Then, at your leisure, you may reread and rethink the incident to detect evidences of ambivalence. When there is a question in your mind, you can give the description of a single segment to someone else for determination or discuss it to get another point of view. You can then use the checklist to make a record of ambivalent behaviors from your original record. The checklist becomes the document you use as a reference for planning to change and as a basis for comparing your behaviors from time to time.

3. *Planned Feedback from Patients*

In all the struggles to develop more effective nurse/patient relationships, few people ever remember that the patient can play a significant part in the process. Since the patient is a party to the relationship, it is folly not to have the data—about his feelings and his perception of situations—that may complement, corroborate, or contradict the nurse's data.

There are useful strategies for obtaining such information from the patient, but their use has limitations, of course, dependent upon how sick he is. One way is direct, giving the patient an opportunity to respond to a question about how he feels. You might first prepare a brief description of a behavior, then read it to the patient and ask him, "Is this an accurate picture of me?" (The description might take the form of one of the case studies in this chapter, with the changes necessary to make it relevant to your own situation and your own behavior.)

The patient must be assured that you are seriously trying to analyze your own behavior as a part of your professional growth. There is no guarantee, however, that the patient will feel free enough to answer candidly. Perhaps if there were three or four patients confronted with the description and the questions at the same time, they might feel safe and respond more freely.

Depending on whether you get a yes or a no answer, you might follow up with additional questions:

FOR A YES ANSWER: Do I often do this or have you noticed it only once? Are there other things I do that remind you of this? Can you describe them? How did it make you feel when I did this?

FOR A NO ANSWER: Have I ever done something similar to this—something that this reminds you of? Can you describe it? How did it make you feel?

A less direct, but nonetheless effective, strategy for getting patient feedback is to give a description of behavior and ask: "Is this what nurses generally are like?"

If the answer is yes, you might follow up with: "Can you tell me some experiences you have had that this reminds you of?"

Again, if you have a group of ambulatory patients who are not very sick, and are probably bored with their stay in the hospital, you might raise the questions and then step back and let them discuss among themselves, while you just listen.

If you would like a more formal feedback process, reword the items in the "Checklist of Ambivalent Behaviors" so that the patient will have no difficulty in answering, and just go down the list asking him the questions and recording his responses. Item 1 might be changed to read: I keep telling you that you ought to learn how to change your position, but every time you start to move I yell at you. Item 2 might be changed to read: I keep telling you to learn your exercises, but when you try, I say you're taking longer to learn than the children downstairs.

Here, again, if there is some doubt that the patient feels comfortable enough to respond in such personal terms, the items may talk about patients "in general" and nurses "in general."

In another book [2] I suggested an indirect strategy for getting information from children through the use of comic strips. The strategy can be adapted for old people (although, of course, there are many adults who respond to the lure of comics) by using other kinds of drawings or photographs. Have a series of pictures showing a nurse and an old patient in poses that suggest quick changing of behaviors and feelings. Ask the person to say what he thinks the two are saying to each other. Or you may have a single picture of a nurse and an old patient suggesting some confusion and ask: "What do you think the nurse in this picture is like?" or "How do you think the patient in this picture feels?"

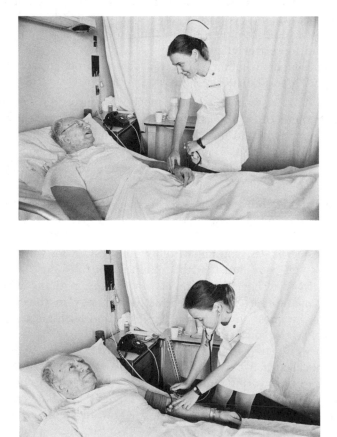

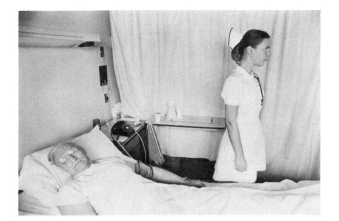

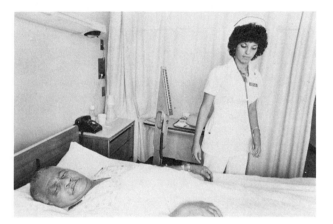

Townsend Wentz

As with most projective techniques, you may get some information you did not set out to get, but, taken all together, you may end up with a body of data from a number of patients that will be helpful to you in self-analysis.

The technique that is always useful is role playing. Here two patients may play patient and nurse, or you and a patient may reverse roles. The person playing the nurse is instructed to act the way a nurse does when he: comes into a room; changes a dressing; tries to teach you something new; is in a good mood; tries to be friendly.

Notes

1. Part of an interview from Charlotte Epstein, *Nursing the Dying Patient,* Reston Publishing Company, Reston, Va., 1975, p. 92.

2. Epstein, op. cit.

3

attitudes and behaviors
toward aging and the aged

stereotyping

Some Instances and Effects

I have often heard Americans say, almost wistfully, how great Orientals are in their attitudes toward the aged, cherishing their wisdom and honoring their lives. Inevitably, they make the comparison with our own culture: we neglect our old people. We are a youth-oriented culture, and so we do not value our old people. We are afraid of growing old, so we do everything to obscure the inevitability of aging.

It is possible that all the time we have accepted the idea that the nuclear family pattern is our norm, we really have not ever gotten away from the extended family pattern. For many of us, grandparents are inextricably bound up with our lives, first living near the nuclear family, and then in later life becoming part of the same household. Just as we are not very clear about our own feelings toward the old, we are not very clear about what the situation really is in the broad social picture.

All of this vagueness in the popular consciousness and this self-denigration seem to be a function of our ambivalence. Many of us live with our aged relatives, but we believe that we, as a nation, do not. We love them, but we think our fellow countrymen do not. We appreciate what they have lived through, yet on a national level we do not think we can learn from them. We admire the active and capable among them, but we insist that, capable or not, they must relinquish their meaningful work at a certain age. We want to live longer, but we begrudge the money for study and treatment of the problems of the aged. We know that the old people who are close to us are unique individuals, with all the individuality that people at every age have, yet we perceive the aged "as a group" in unrealistic and inaccurate ways.

Researchers have warned that, in the study of attitudes about the aged, one must beware of confusing cultural ideas and actual behavior.[1] Such confusion may also be part of the general ambivalence: an inadequate attempt to synthesize what we are with what we think we ought to be.

"The most pervasive view to be found in the literature is that age prejudice exists, presumably for the same reasons that other prejudices occur. . . . Indeed, the correlations with authoritarianism and other measures of discrimination may tentatively support this view."[2] Not only are old people "viewed more negatively than other age groups, [but] old people themselves tend to believe the negative stereotypes attributed to their age group. . . ."[3]

Not many people will venture to deny the obviously deleterious effects of stereotyping racial, religious, and nationality groups. Many Black children have grown up with doubts about their own worth because they have been so bombarded with white perceptions of them as inferior. Jewish youngsters often suffer from a fear of being identified as Jewish, Poles are denigrated in the name of humor, and thousand of Latino children are shunted off into classes for the retarded because they do not communicate in English.

The effects of overgeneralization on old people, however, are less universally recognized, largely because we are, as a society, still engaged in the process of seeking to justify our misconceptions. We find nothing to anger us in the comic routine of a popular TV personality:

INTERVIEWER: What do you think you will be doing in forty years?

COMEDIENNE: Oh, the same thing I'm doing now, except that I'll look like this. (*hunches over, simulating age and decrepitude*)

The audience laughs delightedly at the joke. It is not, after all, an injustice to seventy-year-olds, because isn't that what actually happens to us when we get old? The comedienne is merely being honest and—probably—brave, in admitting that this is her inevitable future. That it is a future of ugliness and incompetence may be regrettable, but, since it is some time off for her, she can still laugh at the picture. *Because it is herself she is laughing at,* not the seventy-year-olds in the audience. (Very few people wonder why the old people don't laugh. Maybe the loss of sense of humor is one of the infirmities of old age!)

One "comedic" routine, apparently a favorite of audiences, is the scene of two old people, sitting in rocking chairs, saying nothing and doing nothing. The scene goes on and on, with the chairs going back and forth, the two old faces expressionlessly carried along by the momentum. It finally becomes clear to some of the people in the audience that this is all there is to the routine, and they begin to laugh. As the awareness grows, the laughter spreads, until the audience is virtually hysterical at the scene—two old people rocking mindlessly into the sunset.

This is quite consistent with the whole process of stereotyping and scapegoating that has victimized other groups in our society. We have, historically, forced certain groups of people into unproductive behaviors, and then we have attributed those behaviors to some innate determinism. We have refused to educate Chicano children, and have relegated them to classes for the retarded. Then we identify Chicanos as intellectually inferior. We have forced Black people to assume menial roles in the labor market, and then have insisted that they were genetically unable to perform at higher levels. With old people, we are doing exactly the same thing: forcing them to sit idly waiting for death, while we insist that this is all they *can* do.

The Jew who told anti-Semitic jokes, or the Black men who encouraged whites to laugh at their portrayals of caricatures of Black people, have, as their ultimate argument against charges of bigotry: "I can't be prejudiced. I'm one myself!" In a curious way, we seem to resist recognizing our own prejudice against old people by implying: "I can't be prejudiced; I'm going to be one myself some day!"

It is certain that there is one riposte we cannot make to our accusers. Most of us cannot contend that "some of my best friends are old people." It sometimes seems as if old people are as effectively segregated from the mainstream of American life as forced unemployment, nursing homes, golden age communities, fear, and disgust can manage. Consider the following experience of a young teacher of kindergarten-age children.

She had, as a child and young woman, been fortunate in having a loving grandmother who lived in the house next to hers and later in a room on the first floor of the same house. From her grandmother, she learned about the time when horses and wagons made up the street traffic, and the iceman delivered blocks of ice, hauling them on his shoulder to each icebox in the neighborhood. She caught some of the excitement of sitting around the first crystal set in the neighborhood. Above all, what characterized their relationship—the very old woman and the child—was an uncritical acceptance of each other. They appreciated each other's need to talk, and could sit in companionable silence when one or the other preferred to sit quietly. The child's sorrows were eased by being held closely; the old woman's were submerged in the delight of having this child so near.

When her grandmother died, Barbara was twenty years old. It was her first experience with the death of someone she loved, and she grieved profoundly. She continued to feel the awful loss even when, as time went on, she began to feel grateful for the time they had had together, and the richness it had added to her life.

When Barbara became a teacher, she found herself in a school in an upper-middle-class area. The four- and five-year-olds in her class knew no old people. They were surrounded with youth and health. Their grandmothers wore miniskirts and bleached the gray from their hair. Their grandfathers were as active as their fathers.

She decided to enlist the aid of some 70- and 80-year-olds that she knew to work in the classroom with her. She wanted to help the children get that sense of continuity of life that she had had as a child. She wanted them to hear firsthand the experiences of a generation that had lived in a fantastically different world. She wanted the children to see the very old as kind and loving and caring.

When the parents of the children heard about her plans for bringing in old people, they were horrified. There really is no other word that accurately describes their reaction. There was almost universal agreement that "It will be bad for the children." When pressed for reasons, they were sure that the children would be frightened. (Their own fear could hardly be contained!) They asked questions that were not questions at all, but clear statements revealing the stereotype they held of old people: "Are they senile?" "Are they clean?" "Do they have communicable diseases?"

When she suggested taking the children to a home for the aged, the parents were beside themselves with anxiety. She persisted in presenting her plan and the rationale for it. Finally, she was permitted to make the arrangements for the visit. But the admonitions were firm: "I don't want them kissing the children." "I don't want them to eat anything there." "They shouldn't be forced to stay if they don't want to." "Just a few minutes is long enough to be there."

Barbara regretted that the frightened parents didn't see the smiles of delight at the children's singing, and the children's smiles of pride at the reception they got. She was sorry that they never saw their children sit rapt at the stories of another age. She hoped one day they would come and feel the beauty of the picture made by a tired child with his head against the knee of an old man and the shaking hand resting lightly on that trusting head.

Our hope for changing the pattern of attitudes and behaviors toward old people may very well lie in the very young, who may still be able to profit from education. But one must not assume that the very young have no negative attitudes, though the common, rather sentimental, belief is that children are not prejudiced—against racial groups, or people who are different, or against old people. In one research designed and instituted some years ago to do a longitudinal study of healthy older people, the researchers got some very clear results: "We had, then, firmly established the fact that children as young as four years old were well able to distinguish the old from the young and that they held marked preferences for people who were not yet old, despite the fact that they might like a particular grandparent." [4]

They also found that the young people they questioned (those four-year-olds who get older) generally reported attitudes that were "scarcely conducive to friendship between the generations." They believed that old people resented them. The old people being studied, however, "expressed no such resentment of the young, but cited rejection, lack of concern and references to age as the things they most resented." [5]

These young adults believed that work for the old was "too strenuous, tiring, distasteful, difficult . . . entirely too much for them." By the old people, however, "the importance of work was seen as having equal significance to the man who is old as to the man who is young. Nearly three-fourths of the older people stressed the psychological value of work and none made reference to its difficulty for those in late age." [6]

There is a curious attitude often revealed about old people that never ceases to surprise me. It is manifested by individuals at every educational level and at various levels of intergroup sensitivity. They believe that old people inevitably have prejudices against other groups and fears of those groups.

One woman, a Roman Catholic nun, offered a friend of hers some help. "If you ever get stuck," she said, "and you need someone to stay with your father, I'll be glad to do it."

"Oh, that's really nice of you. I do appreciate the offer."

"It's not an empty offer, you know. I mean it. It would be no trouble at all. I live not far from you."

"You're a dear. I'll remember that if I'm ever in a bind."

"There's just one thing, though. I don't know . . . I may frighten him." The nun looked troubled, and a little sad.

"Frighten him?"

"Well, you know. . . ."

Suddenly, the light!

"Do you mean he would be afraid of you because you're a nun?"

"Well, I don't necessarily have to wear my habit."

"Oh, really! Where did you ever get an idea like that?"

"Are you sure he won't be disturbed when he sees me?"

This is the kind of question I have never heard anyone ask about people of other ages. As a matter of fact, the pervasive drive in our society is to deny that *anyone ever* would object to another person because of his race or religion. Certainly, if people are aware of the existence of intergroup prejudice, they would not think of asking a mother, for example, if her child is afraid of nuns. Or asking a husband if his wife is afraid of nuns. But, apparently, it is perfectly all right to ask a daughter if her father has such a fear—that is, if her father is 80 years old.

Another instance of this sort of assumption and question involved a professional social worker. She was talking to the daughter of a prospective participant in her local senior citizens' program. The social worker was a white, middle-aged lady serving her witness here on earth by working in a Black neighborhood. She told the old man's daughter, "All my clients are colored. Your father may not want to come here." She said it as if she were quite sure that he would not want to come to play cards and chess and have lunch occasionally with the other old people.

The daughter was moved to gentle sarcasm. "*You* don't seem to mind it," she suggested.

"Oh, this is my *job*."

Apparently socializing is different—as it probably is for most whites in this country. Although I wonder how many young and middle-aged white people this social worker asked, "Do you mind associating with Black people?" Again, the pressure in this country is to deny existence of prejudice. To ask such a question in all likelihood would be viewed as insulting.

It seems to me that the most bizarre aspect of providing services for the aged lies in the assumption that old people constitute some kind of homogeneous group. What is almost completely ignored is that a person's pattern of behavior quite naturally continues throughout his life. To take thousands of individuals with varieties of personalities and life-styles and write programs into which all of them are supposed to fit *just because they are all old* is carrying stereotyping to ludicrous ends!

At one senior citizens' center, eight men ranging in age from 77 to 81 sat around a table trying to respond to the enthusiastic prompting of a young woman.

"Now, you'll enjoy this, you really will! You just follow my directions—it's easy, you'll see! And when you're finished, you'll have a wallet —a *real leather* wallet! You'll like that, won't you?"

Two of the men fingered the bits of leather in front of them. Two others looked at each other quizzically, careful to say nothing that would hurt the feelings of this pleasant young woman. The others looked at her patiently, waiting, as they had learned to wait in the years since their retirement, for other people to get through their "managing." A little while and this one, too, would tire of her association with the elderly. Her enthusiasm would wane gradually, and she would drift away to other jobs and other enthusiasms.

In our conversation later, she referred to herself as a "recreation therapist." Her credentials consisted of a bachelor's degree in elementary education and six years of experience teaching small children. (I got the distinct impression that the kids never were too crazy about her projects, either!)

The center was in an area of the city where most of the men were engaged in blue-collar jobs. Some of the wives worked, often part-time, in garment factories. The adults' day generally was spent working and then relaxing in front of the TV set. When pressed, the women might answer that their hobbies were cooking and taking care of the children. The men's hobbies were TV and drinking beer with their friends.

Most of the old people in the neighborhood continued to live in the homes where they had reared their children. When one spouse died, the other remained alone for a while, and then moved in with a married son or daughter or into an apartment or rooming house. Their time, now that there was no work to go to, was spent largely in visiting with family members and the few friends who were still within walking distance. The center was opened to provide a place in which some of these old people could spend some time, presumably when there was no one to visit with at home, and nothing else to do.

Once in the center—in which they had to become "members," for a small fee—they suddenly found themselves caught up in a program. Although the program projected for the year was announced, with fanfare and printed brochures, as a well-balanced one of creative activities, health seminars, exercise classes, and group singing, the realization never quite matched the projection.

Because some of the activities were offered by volunteers, they never lasted very long. Dances were half-learned, and health seminars never got beyond the exhortations to eat balanced meals. The center was awash with incomplete pieces of petit point and scrapbooks with only a page or two filled.

Other activities run by paid staff were postponed or abandoned when there was an important meeting of community leaders to attend, or a fund-raising drive to manage. Occasionally, an activity even had to be aborted when a staff member needed to find emergency help for one of the old people.

The net effect was a rather sad operation. People wandered in and out of the center. Sometimes the published program was held, more often it was not, so there was no group that came regularly. In a dim corner of the center, there were usually four or five old men playing cards, resisting all the sporadic attempts to get them to participate in the "organized" part of the center's offerings. (The attempts got firmer as the year went on and fewer and fewer people showed up for the scheduled activities.)

Through it all, various community leaders, social workers, and a geriatric physician pointed with pride to the building that housed the center. At the barest hint of encouragement, they would tell you of the difficulties they had encountered in getting the money to buy that building, and the continuing difficulties in getting public and private *monies* for the day-to-day operation. ("Monies," a "professional" word, never used by those of us who only work for a living and never need to scramble for those vast sums that ultimately are used to pay us our salaries.)

And through it all, the staff of the center continued to grow: first a social worker, then two group leaders, then a receptionist, and a secretary, and a student to help. A driver who ran errands for the staff, and someone to manage the volunteers. Until, on any given day, the staff outnumbered the members.

Just as suddenly and totally as the neighborhood of old people were "programmed," they were abandoned. In the summer, virtually all center activity ceased. I never could understand why this happened, since the staff, except for the one or two people on vacation, continued to draw salaries. The old people certainly remained in the neighborhood. Seeing them sitting in front of their houses, I was reminded of the pattern of the school year that persisted long after the reason for it had disappeared into history: ten months of school and two months of vacation, even if there were no crops to plant or harvest. So, for part of June, all of July and August, and part of September, the old people in the neighborhood take a vacation from all the activities they are thought to need so desperately the rest of the year.

Self-Check on Beliefs About Aging

It seems useful to start a detailed discussion of the available data on age and aging by identifying a number of areas where misinformation is widespread and generally accepted without question as accurate. The self-check and the discussions that follow deal with the results of research in the field and focus on facts about aging as well as the facts about responses to aging.

1. In the columns on the right, check True or False for each of the following items.
2. After you have completed the "Self-Check," discuss your answers with the rest of the class (or group) and make some notes on the nature of the arguments advanced for holding the beliefs checked.
   The "Checklist of Arguments" following the "Self-Check" may be useful for identifying some of the bases of the points of view advanced.
3. Do not read the section "Some Data on Age and Aging," which follows "Discussing and Annotating the Self-Check," until after you have discussed and annotated your self-checks.

Self-Check

	True	False

1. Old people get sick and die, not because they are old and worn out but because there are diseases that science does not yet know how to cure.
   Many apparently age-related deficiences in memory and physical functioning may be caused by social isolation and neglect, or by a failure to apply the same kind of diagnostic and remedial knowledge to the aged as is applied to the young.

2. A natural concomitant of old age is the tendency to maintain old values and resist new ideas.

3. Old people often withdraw from interaction with others by pretending to be deaf.

4. A part of old age is overconcern with bodily functions, irritability, and a lack of interest in people and things. There's really nothing much to be done about this besides understanding it for what it is.

5. You cannot expect old people to develop new skills or get involved in learning new things. After all, intelligence, like other functions, naturally declines with old age.

6. Most old people are not interested in the kinds of marital relationships that are of concern to young people.

7. There is no reason to believe that old people need careful supervision because they are more likely to display behaviors that are socially undesirable.

8. It is better to avoid talk about old age with people who are old.

9. By the time an individual reaches old age, he has generally accepted its inevitability and has suitably adjusted his attitudes, values, and behaviors.

Checklist of Arguments

This checklist is to be used during the discussion of the responses to the true–false statements in the "Self-Check." In the appropriate column, briefly write the argument as it occurs in the discussion, and check the source, as given or implied by the speaker. If the group prefers, you may ask two or three people to act as annotators during the discussion. They alone may then use this checklist and share the results of their observations at the conclusion of the discussion.

The Argument	Nobody really knows	Specific, systematic research	Everyone knows	I know a person who exemplifies the rule	They're all that way	The law says so	Authorities say so	He (she) is an exception to the rule

Discussing and Annotating the Self-Check

Here is a transcript of one discussion, annotated to point out clues to the sources of errors. The discussants were a class of eight student nurses who had just completed the "Self-Check." How many such clues were you able to identify in your own and your colleagues' statements during the discussion of your true/false responses?

Discussion by Student Nurses	Clues to Sources of Arguments
STUDENT A: Well, one thing I'm sure about, that no one can argue with: When people get old they just don't funtion as well as they used to.	
STUDENT B: That's true. Even if they don't have a specific medical problem, old people	

Discussion by Student Nurses

just don't have the energy
and stamina that young people have.

STUDENT A: We wouldn't have
mandatory retirement if this
weren't true. People can't
keep working all their lives.
They sort of run down.[1]

(*murmur of laughter*)

STUDENT C: My grandmother was
very active until the day she
died. She was 80 years old
and she actually went to
work every day. She had a
small store that she ran all
by herself after my grandfather died.

STUDENT A: That's marvelous. Of
course, there's always the exception [2] that proves the
rule.

STUDENT D: My grandfather is 92,
and he's still building furni-
ture for the house. He's got
a workroom in the basement
and he's always down there.

STUDENT B: That's wonderful. It's
great if they're able to do
that. It makes it easier on
everybody.

STUDENT E: Oh, I don't know
about that. My mother has
been trying for years to get
my grandmother to slow
down. She's 73, and she insists on taking the subway
every morning to that community center.

STUDENT F: Well, she needs some

Clues to Sources of Arguments

[1] CLUE: The reasoning here is not
unusual: we look at what
we do as a society, and we
give *that* as the justification
for doing it. That is, *because*
we do it, it must be right.

[2] CLUE: If people believe something about a whole group,
each individual of that group
who does not substantiate
the belief is believed to be
an exception. Thus, the
woman car mechanic is the
exception to the rule that
women are genetically non-
mechanical. The Black person who cannot dance is the
exception to the rule that
Black people are born able
to dance and sing.

No matter how many such
"exceptions" are noticed,
the stereotype remains:
"They've all got rhythm."

Discussion by Student Nurses	Clues to Sources of Arguments

recreation. If she can get there all right, why shouldn't she have a place where she can meet her friends?

STUDENT E: It's not recreation. She works there! She helps cook the noon meal, and she helps dish it up.

STUDENT F: Oh.

STUDENT E: My mother just thinks she's worked hard enough all her life. It's time she relaxed and took it easy.

STUDENT G: After a certain age, people have the right to take it easy. They shouldn't feel that they have to keep proving themselves.[3]

STUDENT E: That's what we keep telling my grandmother. But she's so stubborn! She does just what she feels like doing, no matter what anyone says!

STUDENT F: There's a patient like that in the hospital. He's in for tests and he's so edgy. He keeps bothering everyone about when he can go home —because he does some kind of work that he's got to get back to.[4] And he's 68 years old! I'm sure he's retired! But he just can't relax!

STUDENT E: It's not a question of relaxing—it's just stubbornness. That's the way they are —inflexible. You know what they say—You can't teach an old. . . . (*embarrassed laugh*)

[3] CLUE: If we hold a stereotype of a group of people, we may actually become the agents for compelling those people to conform to our image of them. If we expect old people to be unable to work, then we use all kinds of pressures to ensure that our expectations are fulfilled. "You shouldn't work," we say to an old person who wants to work, "You *know* you're not doing it because you *want* to; only because you feel you *have* to. Well, I won't let you do that to yourself. I insist that you relax and *enjoy* the fruits of your lifetime of labor."

If the old person submits to the pressure, then we feel comfortable: "See? I *knew* she was only driving herself because she thought it was expected of her! She's finally convinced that we

Discussion by Student Nurses

I don't really mean that. You can't change them.[5] It's just —you know—old people are a little rigid.

STUDENT G: I don't see people *our* age changing that easily! [6]

STUDENT E: Have you ever tried to change the mind of an older person?! I *know* how impossible it is! [7]

STUDENT G: No—but I have tried to change the mind of a *younger* person!
(*general laughter*)

STUDENT A: I think we can all agree—older people live in the past. It's only natural. That's where their lives are. They're not very interested in young people—or what they think.[8]

Clues to Sources of Arguments

want her to take it easy." Teachers fall into the same kind of trap when they are confronted with children that they expect will not achieve in school: "I teach in the ghetto, you know. Those poor kids—nobody cares about them. How can I expect them to learn when they get no encouragement from home?" So the teacher doesn't teach them, and, of course, the children don't learn, thus fulfilling the teacher's expectation and justifying the continuation of her behavior.

[4] CLUE: One rarely communicates with another person about his work without getting clear on what kind of work the person is engaged in. This type of reference to the patient's work seems to indicate that student F assigns very little importance to work that a man of his age can do. This is consistent with the cultural expectations that a man retires from the significant work of his life at 65. After that, he is encouraged to do volunteer work, or puttering of one kind or another, activity that is supposed to provide meaningful involvement for a person who has just been deprived of his meaningful

Discussion by Student Nurses	Clues to Sources of Arguments

Clues to Sources of Arguments

work. It becomes clear that the protestations that post-retirement work makes valuable contribution to society is not really believed by *this* young person, at least.

[5] CLUE: Student E seems to be speaking out of a combination of belief in the prevailing stereotype of old people and an on-going experience she is having with one old person. From what we know of the development of stereotypic thinking, it is likely that the belief that old people are rigid and resistant to change came first, and functions as the basis for her perception of the old person she knows.

Because that person's behavior does not conform with her wishes, it is perceived, in terms of the stereotype, as the rigidity of age. It is likely that similar behavior in a young person would be perceived as idiosyncratic—that is, as the stubbornness of this particular person, or merely the presentation of an opposing point of view.

[6] CLUE: It is interesting to see how an attempt by student G to introduce a broader perspective for consideration is

[7] CLUE: countered by evidence of a single experience as proof

Discussion by Student Nurses	Clues to Sources of Arguments
	of the stereotype. Student G's persistence is met with laughter—(the laughter of recognition?)—but is
	[8] CLUE: ignored by student A, who actually believes that there is no disagreement with her point of view.
	Deducing from experimental data on dealing with overt expression of prejudice, we suggest that this kind of projection, believing that everybody agrees with you, can be offset by direct statements of opposition to the view. The oblique, half-joking protests of student G are more easily blocked from perception, and the meaning of the general laughter can be interpreted as being sympathetic to the stereotypic thinker.

Some Data on Age and Aging [7]

In the following observations and reports of research on each true–false item, it becomes clear that although the research is meager and much of it is inconclusive, one beacon light stands out: people would do well to concentrate on trying to relate to the aged as if they were sometimes interesting, sometimes dull, sometimes loving, sometimes hateful, men, friends, enemies, and parents—in short, unique individuals with whom it is interesting to establish and build relationships.

In making a distinction between the old and the aged, Ivan Illich says, "The old run around and the aged are institutionalized." [8] What he is saying, it seems to me, is that the term "the aged" has become a label for implying that old people are mostly alike, and can be studied and treated as if their individual differences were negligible. Most old people

—like most middle-aged and young people—"run around," that is, they defy pat generalizations about them.

It occurs to me that, as old people more and more realize their political strength through vocal organization, the generalizations will slowly give way to more realistic bases for social planning.

1. There is a pervasive hopelessness about old age that seems to be a function of confusing its inevitability with all the negative concomitants that we attribute to it. That is, because we know that old age is unavoidable, we seem to believe that all the things we don't like about it are also inevitable. As a result, old people and their families are often resigned to living with debilities that, in a younger person, would be vigorously diagnosed, treated, and, perhaps, even cured. As a result, too, our national commitment to research on aging is miniscule, especially when we put it up against the awesome fact that almost all of us stand to benefit directly at some time from the findings of such research.

There is no reason to believe that the age range within which most of us die cannot be significantly raised if we traded our attitudes of resignation and hopelessness for belief in the equal worthwhileness of treating and curing people of all ages.

Curtis defines aging as an increasing probability of contracting one of the degenerative diseases. Just what is at the bottom of this increasing probability is likely a complex, multistep process that involves more than one biological mechanism.[9] The point to be made for living is that we do not die of old age. We die of disease, sometimes of disease that science does not yet know how to treat. But sometimes, because the younger people think we have lived along enough.

This attitude is not as conscious as that statement makes it seem. On the contrary, even old people in medical crisis are shocked awake and tubed for maintenance. But the attitude is apparent every time a physician says, "What can you expect? You're seventy years old!" Every time an orthopedist says, "How much walking do you have to do? You're 75 years old!" Every time treatable illness is overlooked because the expectation is that the observable symptoms are merely signs of old age. "Frequently . . . the older patient is responded to as 'hopeless' from a medical point of view and is seen as operating with machinery that is worn out, with symptoms relating primarily to his age. . . . It is important to realize that we are dealing with a potentially valuable person who, while more likely to have a disease than a younger adult, is not diseased merely by virtue of his years." [10]

2. When we stop to realize that a man of eighty today has lived through—*and adjusted to*—innovations that were in the realm of fantasy scarcely one hundred years ago, we must reject the concept that old people cannot live adequately with new ideas.

If older people seem often to value things that are out of date, it may be the case of a culture causing the phenomenon and then blaming the victim for exhibiting it. This is done with our attitude toward the very poor, who are victims of a society that reinforces and perpetuates poverty, especially in its approach to schooling, and then blames poor people for their condition.

In isolating the aged from other age groups, in reinforcing the idea that one must "act his age," in keeping older people from involvement in activities that necessitate changes in behaviors and attitudes, our society leaves older people alone with the remnants of their past. Then we maintain that clinging to the past is a natural function of old age.

However, in spite of the pressures to live in the past, the stereotype of old people as politically conservative needs some reconsideration.[11]

> Twentieth century America has been marked by a growing liberalism in social and political philosophy. Each generation appears somewhat more liberal than preceding ones. But this trend . . . is subject to reversal if social conditions change. . . . In a comparative study at a midwestern university . . . contemporary students are [shown to be] ideologically more conservative than their parents. . . . Conceivably, in forty years when they are both old, the depression generation which reached adulthood under Roosevelt and the New Deal would be socially and politically more liberal than the post-war generation which came of age under Eisenhower. . . . Conservative values are *not* attributable to aging per se.

Religious belief, which is often considered an aspect of conservatism, is also a facet of the stereotype of old age. But the data on this do not exist. "There is no evidence to substantiate the stereotype that people actually become more religious as they age. And there is impressive evidence that they systematically share many basic beliefs of the younger generations, including consumption preferences, social mobility, values, images of the good life, and others."[12]

3. Because we are handicapped in our view of the old by our prejudices, we are quick to ascribe to old age personality traits that may very well be caused by physical problems that would be quickly detected and treated if a younger person were the one suffering. For example, ". . . men who appear to be rigid and angry, indeed, crotchety and mean . . ." may be suffering from a hearing loss.[13]

Recruitment deafness is the disease that is the subject of an old and constantly repeated joke about old people, used to reinforce the stereotype that the old are cantankerous and difficult to live with just because they are old. With this kind of deafness, normal speech cannot be heard, but shouting is heard as shouting, so the sufferer is forever complaining that people are either whispering to him or yelling at him. Because of the apparent inconsistencies in response, the younger person's conclusion may be that the older person is faking, turning his deafness on and off as it suits him. Even sophisticated researchers of the factors of aging have come to this conclusion. Here, again, the belief that an old person's behavior is attributable merely to old age can actually function as a self-fulfilling prophecy, causing those very behaviors that we expect old people to demonstrate.

"Don't mind grandpa, he's just old," may very well begin to make grandpa believe that everyone is conspiring against him, and that will merely reinforce the idea that the problem is senility. Indeed, in one series of studies "it was found that the single most important variable which related to overall level of deterioration was hearing loss." [14]

It is likely that such traits as stubbornness, touchiness, grouchiness, attributed to old people—if they exist at all—are often results of untreated illnesses or the effects of improper drug use. "Government drug abuse officials told Congress that they are concerned about the overprescribing of tranquilizers, sedatives and hypnotic drugs to create so-called 'chemical straitjackets' among nursing home patients. [But] 'underutilization of drugs with the elderly was far more prevalent and consequential . . .' according to Dr. Bertram S. Brown, director of the National Institute of Mental Health." This was corroborated by "Dr. Robert I. DuPont, director of the National Institute on Drug Abuse, [who] said underuse of drugs can result from aged persons taking drugs improperly, lacking money for necessary drugs or transportation to health care facilities, and having difficulty opening containers." [15]

Dr. Morton Ward, medical director of the Philadelphia Geriatric Center, which operates a comprehensive mental and physical health screening program for the aged, says that about one out of six patients screened so far has been suffering from some undiagnosed, treatable illness. The ailments range from brain tumors and diabetes to extensive heart damage.[16]

4. Kastenbaum suggests that *"many of the negative patterns of behavior we tend to associate with old age are the result of a bereavement overload."* [17] Too many friends and loved ones die too quickly; a home and possessions are sold; faculties are diminished or lost. A younger person, faced with a number of losses following quickly one upon the other might help himself by becoming absorbed in his work or other activities—which the old person cannot do. The results may be over-concern with bodily functions, reluctance to become involved with people or care for things, suicide or neglect of self, irritability and bitterness.

"All of the negative reactions that have been catalogued above are observed in those elderly people whom we usually consider to be suffering from the general effects of old age. But we now have an alternative explanation, namely, that the adverse changes exist in consequence of multiple bereavements, not because of some mysterious and immutable transformation that occurs as a direct consequence of aging." [18]

In a longitudinal study of fifty-nine people, 70 years old, relatively advantaged and healthy, Neugarten, Havighurst, and Tobin report:[19]

> There is considerable evidence that, in normal men and women, there is no sharp discontinuity of personality with age, but instead an increasing consistency. Those characteristics that have been central to the personality seem to become even more clearly delineated, and those values the individual has been cherishing become even more salient. In the personality that remains integrated—and in an environment that permits—patterns of overt behavior are likely to become increasingly consonant with the individual's underlying personality needs and his desires.

It would seem that such consistency signals a development toward greater mental health in old age—again, if the individual is permitted to develop free of the pressures to fragment his life to conform to societal expectations of the aged.

5. Although many researchers have found that "functional capacities decline with advancing age," [20] one must continue to be wary of accepting the implications that are sometimes advanced. For example, Hrachovec continues the observation, "some of them go faster in one person than in another, whether involving the heart, kidney, respiratory function, muscular strength, memory, or learning capacities." He goes on to present experimental data on physical capacities but no information at all on memory or learning capacities. Few people, including scientists, seem immune from the ". . . widespread assumption that intelligence normally declines in advanced adulthood and old age." [21] (I take for granted here that learning and memory are functions of intelligence, although the space needed to outline the difficulties of defining intelligence goes beyond the scope of this discussion.)

Baltes and Schaie, departing from the traditional research method of comparing different age groups at a single point in time, tested people at different times in their lives with a variety of instruments designed to get at different components of intellectual functioning. They found that on at least three of the four components, ". . . people of average health can expect to maintain or even increase their level of performance into old age." [22]

Other researchers are beginning to make experimental attempts to improve the intellectual functioning of older people, working on the premise that remediable biological and social factors can directly increase intelligence. Even the speed with which people respond on many tests, usually thought to depend on physical differentials, apparently can be increased by motivational factors (like giving Green Stamps for working faster!)[23]

6. "One of the most important factors influencing the emotional security of the elderly and one of the most neglected areas of research is the marriage and family relationships of the older person." [24]

Since a significant majority of older people are married, research in family relationships would seem logically to concern itself with older marriages, but generally that has not been the case.

There is one study, involving 227 older husbands and wives, in which the researchers identified twenty-four factors on the basis of which they measured marital need satisfaction:[25]

1. Providing a feeling of security in me.
2. Expressing affection toward me.
3. Giving me an optimistic feeling toward life.
4. Expressing a feeling of being emotionally close to me.
5. Bringing out the best qualities in me.
6. Helping me to become a more interesting person.
7. Helping me to continue to develop my personality.
8. Helping me to achieve my individual potential (becoming what I am capable of becoming).
9. Being a good listener.
10. Giving me encouragement when I am discouraged.
11. Accepting my differentness.
12. Avoiding habits which annoy me.
13. Letting me know how he or she really feels about something.
14. Trying to find satisfactory solutions to our disagreements.
15. Expressing disagreement with me honestly and openly.
16. Letting me know when he or she is displeased with me.
17. Helping me to feel that life has meaning.
18. Helping me to feel needed.
19. Helping me to feel that my life is serving a purpose.
20. Helping me to obtain satisfaction and pleasure in daily activities.
21. Giving me recognition for my past accomplishments.
22. Helping me to feel that my life has been important.
23. Helping me to accept my past life experiences as good and rewarding.
24. Helping me to accept myself despite my shortcomings.

These twenty-four factors of significant concern to the subjects do not indicate that needs of older husbands and wives are different from needs of younger husbands and wives. It becomes clear that the drive for continuing personal development, the need for purpose and self-acceptance, the value put on honesty are aspects of a person that do not become extinguished at some arbitrary point signaling the end of "middle age."

Perhaps of equal significance in considering these needs and values is the fact that most older people rely heavily, emotionally and materially, on their relationships with their adult offspring. There are not many important studies that deal with such relationships, but it would appear that these factors may be used to evaluate any intimate relationship between adults.

The point of all this is that there is no reason to suppose that, in their relationships with significant adults in their lives, old people look for satisfactions that are any different from what young people look for.

7. In spite of the popularity at one time of disengagement theory as an explanation of aging, most theorists recognize that, although aging is accompanied by a variety of problems: [26]

> We are now reasonably confident . . . that for most older people the maintenance of a relatively high level of social involvement and activity contributes significantly to a sense of well-being. This remains so even though the level of involvement and activity does characteristically diminish with age. At the same time, we have a new appreciation of the variety of life styles which appear to . . . reflect satisfactory articulation of personal needs with social expectations. Although the motivation to conform socially does appear to weaken in the later years, competent social behavior in a variety of forms nevertheless appears to be the rule among the old.

8. It would seem that our national "dilemma," which Gunnar Myrdal defined as a conflict between our democratic ideals and our pervasive racial prejudice, makes us uncomfortable at any mention of race, unless we are talking only to members of our own race. A similar phenomenon may be observed among those who are not yet old: there seems to be tacit understanding that it is bad form to discuss old age with old people. The feeling is that the old person will in some way be affronted by the mention of age, as if being old is an unmentionable debility—like being black, or wearing leg braces. One must be polite, one must pretend not to notice the flaw, because, after all, people are equal and are entitled to equal treatment.

But it is obvious that the belief in equal treatment is too often not translated into actual equal treatment, a contradiction that we are forever trying to rationalize away, and that makes us so uncomfortable that we do not like to bring it up in the presence of the victimized groups.

Slowly, the victims have been provoked to the realization that *they* must initiate the talk, *they* must bring the awareness of prejudice and discrimination to the national consciousness, they must take the initiative in instituting change. They will no longer permit others to pretend—under a veneer of polite avoidance—that everyone is equal.

9. "[T]he available evidence . . . suggest[s] that many, perhaps the majority, of individuals are ill-prepared to accept the fact of old age. . . . The charge that one fails 'to act one's age' is often leveled at the older persons . . . and the comment that one has or has not 'grown old gracefully' may be a commentary on the inadequacy of socialization to the old age stratum." [27]

It is not surprising that there is resistance to adapting to a condition that is viewed with such confusion and with so much rejection. Mc-Tavish's review of research to 1971 indicates that "Most investigators report findings which support the view that attitudes toward the elderly . . . in industrialized, Western nations . . . [are generally negative]." [28] It is clear too, however, that there are numbers in every study who have strongly positive pictures of old people.

The stereotypes of old people vary, with some people holding one picture of what all old people are like, and other people holding a completely different picture. In a number of investigations of acceptance and rejection of old people [29] one study shows that, although 83 percent of the respondents felt that old people are good to children and 64 percent believed they were kind, 46 percent thought they were stubborn and grouchy. Although 50 percent believed they made friends easily, 35 percent thought they were bossy, 33 percent that they meddle in other people's affairs, 23 percent that they are cranky and hard to get along with, 19 percent that they are grouchy, and 8 percent that they cannot cooperate even on simple tasks.

Another study finds that, although 79 percent agreed that old people like the company of those younger, 73 percent believed they are sometimes inconsiderate of the views of younger persons, 36 percent felt they are annoying, and 77 percent see them as apt to complain. In that same study 92 percent believed that old people are valuable because of their experience (a statistic difficult to reconcile with the 23 percent who responded that old people are poor managers of affairs).

In still another study, 27.7 of the respondents had negative feelings when they were with an old person. Add to this the 38.9 percent who felt passive and subordinate, and we begin to have an idea of the problems we face in efforts to develop a culture free of ageism.

The myths of the extremes flourish everywhere, sometimes in the head of the same person, even though they seem to contradict each other and cancel each other out. At one extreme is the belief that "The very young and the very old reach quick understanding. . . . In some families (or groups or societies or cultures) the old and the young form an alliance within the larger family. For example, I thought my parents extremely dull in experience and life-style compared with my grandparents. I thought they lacked sensitivity and spirit. . . . But with the old people I knew I could relax and enjoy their company and their stories." [30]

At the other extreme is the belief that led to the law in Youngstown, Arizona, that has zoned an area for old people and has made it against the law for any children to live within its boundaries. The implication is that old people and children cannot get along together at all.

The truth about old people, like most truths about all people, lies in the whole range of diversities between the two extremes. The stereotypic extremes of views often result in destructive—and even bizarre—treatment of the old. In daily experiences, in the prescriptions of professionals, and in national policy, old people are buffeted by conflicting messages sent out by a society that is not sure how it feels about aging and the old.

Notes

1. Donald G. McTavish, "Perceptions of Old People: A Review of Research Methodologies and Findings," *The Gerontologist*, Vol. 11, No. 4, Winter, 1971, pp. 99–101.

2. Ibid.

3. Vern L. Bengston, "Inter-age Perceptions and the Generation Gap," *The Gerontologist*, Vol. 11, No. 4, Winter, 1971, pp. 85–89.

4. Natalie Harris Cabot, *You Can't Count on Dying*, Houghton Mifflin Company, Boston, 1961, p. 64.

5. Ibid., p. 68.

6. Ibid., pp. 68–69.

7. Many of the articles cited here have been reprinted in *Perspectives in Aging, I. Research Focus*, edited and compiled by Frances G. Scott and Ruth M. Brewer, Oregon Center for Gerontology, Eugene, Oregon, 1971.

8. Ivan Illich, with Sam Keen, "Medicine Is a Major Threat to Health," *Psychology Today*, May, 1976, pp. 66–77.

9. Howard J. Curtis, "A Composite Theory of Aging," *The Gerontologist*, Vol. 6, No. 3, Part I, September, 1966, pp. 143–149.

10. Carl Eisdorfer, "The Implications of Research for Medical Practice," *The Gerontologist*, Vol. 10, No. 1, Part II, Spring, 1970, pp. 62–67.

11. Irving Rosow, *Social Integration of the Aged*, The Free Press, New York, 1967, p. 12.

12. Ibid., p. 32.

13. Eisdorfer, op. cit.

14. Ibid.

15. *Philadelphia Daily News*, June 10, 1976.

16. *The Philadelphia Inquirer*, May 30, 1976.

17. Robert Kastenbaum, "Death and Bereavement in Later Life," in *Death and Bereavement*, Austin Kutscher, ed., Charles C Thomas, Springfield, Ill., 1969, pp. 28–54.

18. Ibid.

19. Bernice L. Neugarten, Robert J. Havighurst, and Sheldon S. Tobin, "Personality and Pattern of Aging," *Middle Age and Aging*, Bernice L. Neugarten, ed., University of Chicago Press, Chicago, 1968, pp. 173–177.

20. Josef P. Hrachovec, "Health Maintenance in Older Adults," *Journal of the American Geriatrics Society*, Vol. 17, No. 5, May, 1969, pp. 433–499.

21. Paul B. Baltes and K. Warner Schaie, "Aging and IQ; The Myth of the Twilight Years," *Psychology Today*, March, 1974, pp. 35–40.

22. Ibid.

23. Ibid.

24. Nick Stinnett, Janet Collins, and James E. Montgomery, "Marital Need Satisfaction of Older Husbands and Wives," *Journal of Marriage and the Family*, November, 1968, pp. 428–434.

25. Ibid.

26. G. L. Maddox, "Themes and Issues in Sociological Theories of Human Aging," *Human Development*, Vol. 13, No. 1, 1970, pp. 17–27.

27. Ellen Page Robin, "Discontinuities in Attitudes and Behaviors of Older Age Groups," *The Gerontologist*, Vol. 11, No. 4, Winter, 1971, Part II, pp. 79–81.

28. McTavish, op. cit.

29. Ibid.

30. Sharon R. Curtin, *Nobody Ever Died of Old Age*, Little, Brown and Company, Boston, 1972, pp. 45–46.

*exercises in awareness
and skill development*

stereotyping and
its behavioral effects

Affective Discussion

In exploring any subject in which there is a significant emotional investment, time and opportunity must be provided to permit students to express their feelings freely. Without such opportunity, the tendency is—on the part of the instructor—to present information, and—on the part of the student—to memorize that information for the purpose of repeating it on an examination. Although there is some recent evidence that mere learning of facts can change behavior, the overwhelming weight of the evidence indicates that people who have strong emotional commitments to an idea or a set of beliefs are not receptive to new information that goes against those beliefs.

What seems to be needed by those in the process of learning is a chance to pour out the fears and anxieties, the hatreds and ambivalences that have long been bottled up inside them. Learners engaged in this "pouring out":

1. Realize that the feelings they have are not insane or immoral or otherwise reprehensible. They merely exist, and are shared by others.

2. Can begin to examine their feelings objectively, bringing to the examination whatever information they are able to use at that time. The ability to use new information increases, as is evidenced by the increase in quality of discussion as learners continue their involvement in the various exercises.

To ensure free expression, the instructor must refrain from evaluating what is said or interfering in the discussion process. The vital function of the instructor during such a discussion is to diagnose the educational needs that are revealed so that she may provide appropriate experiences to fill these needs.

If there is no instructor in the group, two of the group members may act as observers, in order to record evidence of stereotyping, possible sources of error, and gaps in experience. Such information is then fed back to the group and used as the basis for planning further study. In giving this feedback, it is well to avoid identifying the individuals who made the errors. Such identification is ego threatening and could inhibit future discussions. It is also unnecessary, because it is *the group* that is planning and pursuing the study, and everyone in it will be exposed to the learning experiences.

As study continues, the observations and feedback will become more and more sophisticated, as will the group's reaction to it, until the whole group will be able to detect errors in its own discussions and will need no observers.

There should be no more than eight or nine people in the discussion group, in order to maintain an atmosphere of confidentiality and to provide optimum opportunity for everyone to participate. Fewer than seven people may not provide enough stimulation to keep the discussion going.

Following are questions that are suitable for opening up the subject of age and aging:

1. What Frightens You About Growing Old?

This is the kind of question that would be useful for any age group. Although an assumption is made that everyone in the group has fears about aging, the participants are not really bound to admit fears. Actually, many start by denying that they are afraid, and it is only after others have begun to talk about a fear of being helpless or a fear of being in pain that those who deny feel comfortable enough to explore their own fears.

2. What Do You Hate About Nursing Old People?

Many nurses experience some shock when they hear this question. However, it reassures many of them that such feelings are real and that no one will condemn them for having them. Generally, great relief is felt by the participants that they are free to express such feelings, instead of hiding them and feeling guilty for having them. They begin to discover, also, that opportunity to express the feelings in the relatively safe atmosphere of the accepting, nonevaluating group helps them to keep the feelings from adversely affecting their behavior when they are treating old people.

3. How Do You Think Old People Feel About You?

Generally, the discussion starts out with the disclaimer that one cannot make generalizations about old people—that individual attitudes vary, even among the old. If the instructor says nothing, just waits, participants will begin to relate personal experiences, most of them illustrating that old people really do not like young people very much, do not understand them, and are even sometimes afraid of them. Occasionally, someone will tell about a loving, accepting grandmother or great aunt.

But what slowly becomes apparent in many discussions is the attitude of the participants toward old people, the stereotypes they hold, and the profound wish—and expectation—that they will be different when they are old.

4. How Do Old People and Young People Feel About Each Other?

This is a question suitable for a group formed, perhaps, in a community health center. Some of the old people who come in to be treated and some of the young people—nurses, physicians, social workers, community volunteers—could sit together and begin to establish honest and open communication with each other. Stereotypes are challenged on the spot by individuals most victimized by them, and misconceptions are corrected. Most important, the people whose interaction is vital in the success of the treatment work directly to make that interaction as satisfying and as productive as it can possibly be.

Words and Actions [1]

If one is to develop a degree of empathy with people of other groups, one must first become aware of the errors one accepts as facts about those groups. One must begin to try to understand how one's own behavior often betrays beliefs about groups that hurt and antagonize others— even when one is only minimally aware that he has those beliefs and that he is acting on them.

In the following exercise, participants often start out by insisting that there is really nothing undesirable about the remark they have just made or the behavior they have just employed—that they don't mean anything "wrong" by it. Furthermore, they cannot understand why anyone should be insulted by the words or the action. Even some old people take the same stance at first, but it is not long before they and their younger associates arrive at a higher level of consciousness and begin to question the sources of the comments and behaviors they have become accustomed to take for granted.

Directions for The Exercise

1. Each one of the following items is to be written on a small card:

1. "She's aged so gracefully."
2. "I'm younger, so it's up to me to apologize."
3. "Why doesn't he act his age?"
4. "He's 70 years old, but he's really very sharp."
5. "The women's dresses are on the next floor; this is the misses' department."
6. "He wouldn't enjoy that film; he's 68 years old!"
7. "Don't tell her about Mary; she'll only worry."

8. "I don't think you ought to be out in this weather" (or "up so late," or "drink," or "smoke").
9. Young man bypasses the old people on the street and asks only young people to sign his petition.
10. Young woman motions an old man to leave the elevator ahead of her.
11. Acquaintance talking *about* the old man or woman *to* the younger person with him: "How is he feeling? He looks fine."

2. Seven or eight people sit in a small circle, with the shuffled deck of cards face down on a chair in the center.

3. Next to the cards on the chair have a sphygmomanometer, with the bulb valve tightened, so that when the bulb is pumped, the pressure remains steady.

4. The first person in the circle turns up the top card and reads it aloud.

5. She then pumps the sphygmomanometer three times, to symbolize the building up of pressure in the person who hears or observes what has just been read.

6. Anyone else in the group who is annoyed, or hurt, or angered by the words or the action described on the card may also pump the sphygmomanometer as many times as he wishes.

Even if no one in the group has any negative feeling at hearing the card read, the reader must still pump the sphygmomanometer three times to symbolize such feeling. The point is that these remarks and behaviors imply stereotypes held by the person whose words or behaviors are described on the card, and many people are aware of the destructive effects of stereotyping. The object of the activity is to help everyone in the group to reach that level of awareness.

7. After everyone who wishes to do so has pumped the sphygmomanometer, the group discusses the item on the card, trying to understand why it causes the buildup of negative feelings.

The following discussion of these items may help by providing additional information.

When the group feels that it has explored a card sufficiently, another person reads the next card and follows the same procedure. Not more than five minutes should be spent on a card, lest the activity bog down in argument and repetition and the participants begin to lose interest.

Discussion of The Items

1,3. The implication in this observation seems to be that the old person behaves in ways that are appropriate to her age. It is when one begins to identify these "appropriate" behaviors that the stereotype emerges: It is not appropriate for an old woman to wear clothes that are too obviously fashionable, or to fix her hair in any new fashion unless it has been severely adapted for old women, or to have young (intimate) friends, or to fall in love, or to be an activist for social change. The picture that "growing old gracefully" conjures up is one of sweet and quiet resignation, of withdrawal from self-assertion and vigorous thinking.

Although it is probably true that this kind of behavior suits some old people—and some young people as well—the expectation that it is right for all old people is not only unrealistic but has the effect of forcing old people to comply with the picture. As the following items are discussed, it may become clear how that forcing process operates.

2. There is a condescension here masking as respect that cannot help but make a self-respecting old person angry. The individual seems to be saying, "I am not apologizing because I did you an injustice and wish to beg your pardon; I am apologizing—even though *you* did *me* an injustice—because you are old, and the ordinary expectations between peers are not operative between us."

Thus the old person is put beyond the pale of reasonable expectations in the relationships between people. He is not expected to assume the responsibilities that go along with productive human relations. He does not belong.

4. The stereotype is clear: after people reach a certain age their intellectual functions are severely circumscribed. Old people cannot be expected to think clearly, to perceive accurately. Of course, there are exceptions! *You* are one. But about old people in general, we can safely say that they are no longer with it.

This is the classic formula of the bigot: They are all alike—with some exceptions that prove the rule.

5,9. These are the words and behaviors of strangers, who are making assumptions about an old person on the basis of what they think all old people are like. The saleswoman thinks the dresses in her department are too "youthful" for the woman who has just approached her. Like the salesperson who assumes that the black person cannot afford her wares and that the dungaree-clad person is not to be trusted, the belief that she knows exactly what the people in the group are like is an insult to the individual to whom she is talking.

I have stood in the shelter of a doorway on a busy street and tallied the numbers of people approached by a young man with a petition to get a radical political party on the ballot. He has systematically avoided, walked around, and ignored all gray-haired people, all people who seemed to be older than 25 or 30. His request for signatures only from young people betrayed his belief that only the young were interested in democracy, radical change, and questions of constitutionality. I am sad to say that the sneers and refusals of many of the young people he approached did nothing to change his behavior.

6. Are tastes in films, pictures, books, and other art forms a function of age? It is obviously true that tastes vary in time from generation to generation, and a person who develops his preferences in one generation may view the preferences of another generation with a somewhat jaundiced eye. However, there is a large overlap in taste change, and there are always people in each generation whose tastes and interests are more characteristic of the next or the past generation. To take it for granted that an old person has no taste for new art forms is to make it easier to exclude old people from contemporary social and cultural events. It then becomes necessary to provide events for the "senior citizens," based on some agency director's conception of what old people like, and a whole new professional industry develops around activities for the old. No inconsiderable effort in this industry is expended in convincing old people that they *ought* to attend these special activities, when the effort might be better spent in providing transportation and other help in getting them to the activities the rest of America flocks to.

7. Here is another way in which old people are kept apart from significant relationships by assuming they are unable to cope with the unpleasant realities of life. Whatever evidence we have on the subject indicates that people who have persevered through the assorted vicissitudes of life for six, seven, or eight decades seem to be better able to deal with difficulties, accidents, and tragedies than do many younger people. Instead of drawing on the strength of the experienced in our population, we keep them in a limbo inhabited by all those who are not privy to our secrets.

8,11. Item 8 assumes that all old people need to be protected from their own defective judgment about behaviors that are more dangerous for them than they are for younger people. Not only do they not know enough to come in out of the rain, but rain has terrible consequences for them. In addition, anyone who knows these two facts has a right to advise and/or compel an old person to act on them.

The corollary of this kind of stereotyping is the practice of talking about an old person as if he were not present. We do something similar to children, presuming to advise them, push them, pull them, and, finally, talk about them in their presence as if they were inanimate objects.

It is true that some old people do not hear (in which case we might *write* our communication) or do not understand (in which case we might at least make some human touching gesture while we talk to relatives and guardians). But to assume that the old person here now neither hears nor understands is part of the stereotype of the old.

10. If we expect old people to cling to and value the mores of an earlier age, why are we so quick to violate an old man's dignity by

insisting he precede a woman out of the elevator? Even with the rapid progress in equality between the sexes, most young men have difficulty in changing the pattern of intersex etiquette. Is it possible that the belief that old people are asexual makes this kind of behavior so widespread? The young woman never thinks that the old person's sense of manhood is violated when he is forced to abandon the traditional niceties in his casual relationships with women.

Studying Social Distance: Stereotypes and Friendship Patterns

Generally, many of us protest—sometimes too much—that we are not prejudiced against racial, ethnic, or sex groups. However, when we make our statement about old people, we go far beyond the mere denial of prejudice. We profess love and admiration for their wisdom, compassion and respect for their powers of survival.

We have examined some of the practical evidence that our society's love is somewhat lacking. On an individual basis, sentimentality can be mistaken for love. When confronted with the necessity for interaction with an old person, when old people can no longer be completely avoided, if one is teary enough and uses loving words, it is easy to hide from yourself that there is little love. One person told me:

> My married sister gets misty-eyed whenever she speaks of our father. "He's so old, Flo. Do you remember how tall and straight he used to walk?" And she puts a handkerchief to her nose. She ought to cry less and give more. Oh, I don't mean give material things. She does that, all right. On birthdays and holidays, she comes laden down with presents— embarrassingly laden down. If she happens to be out of town on a birthday, she makes certain to call—first thing in the morning. "I can hardly believe it!" she squeals over the phone to him. "Eighty years old! You're wonderful, Dad. Just wonderful!" And to me, infinitely more sadly, "He's so *old*, Flo!" There's a catch in her voice when she says it.

That sort of thing is about on a par with teachers who *love* children and nurses who *love* people. What this *love* usually consists of is a lot of kissing and hugging and not a few tears; it rarely provides for the needs of the people who are so loved. It offers no patience when learning is difficult, no acceptance when hostility is acted out, no time to listen when fears are overwhelming. What it offers is a dramatic catch in the throat and a heartfelt sigh, while others do what has to be done.

"Don't you just *love* old people?" one young inhalation therapist gushed at me. She was stricken when I said no: I don't love black people, I don't love children, I don't love old people. I love my father, who is old;

I think *all* people are entitled to live their lives as fully as they want to and are able to until the moment they die. I love my friends; I demand that *all* people get every possible opportunity to continue to learn and grow and participate in all the world has to offer. There are people I love —of all ages, and races and relationships to me. But when it comes to my students, love is not the significant factor in our relationship: what they need is my help in learning what they need to function in their professions.

As people grow to adulthood and become more involved in goals and activities apart from their parents, sentimentality may even be used as justification for staying away from parents, especially as they become old. From the experiences with adults whose parents have grown old, it becomes clear that, if we can develop awareness of the way sentimentality obscures the reality of feelings and beliefs and makes us blind to the destructiveness of our behavior, we can make significant strides toward improving relationships between younger people and old people, and consequently providing a better life for all of us as we age.

One man, for example, told his sister who had arranged to have their seventy-year-old mother come and live with her, "I won't come to see you for a while—give Mom a chance to settle in; give you both some time to adjust. But remember, I'm not far away. You're not alone."

The message is that the sentimentalist is really a very sensitive, even empathic, person. *He* knows what his sister needs—what she needs is to be left alone to work out her problems. He doesn't even have to ask what *she* wants, so accurate are his perceptions!

A nurse told me recently, "All the time my father was in the hospital and then recuperating at home, my brother never came to see him. I know he loves his father and really cares what happens to him, but he might just as well never have heard about the broken hip. When the old man was back on his feet my brother told me one day, 'I feel so guilty about not coming to see Pop. But, you know, I don't think I could have taken it. I think seeing him helpless, in the hospital, maybe dying, would have destroyed me. You're more used to the whole business.' "

Can you see what a soft-hearted, *feeling* person he is? He feels so strongly that he can't bear to see his poor old father suffer. (Like the ancient—and bitter—joke about the soft-hearted rich man who exhorted his retinue to keep the poor man out of his sight because he couldn't bear to witness suffering.)

Often sentimentality even attacks the adult offspring who has herself assumed the care of an aged parent.

"How is your father these days?"

"Oh. . . ." (*sad shaking of head*)

"Isn't he well?"

"Yes . . . he's well. . . ." (*deep sigh*)

The message is clear: The poor dear. I've given him a home when he needed one. Color the martyr golden.

Now look at your own behavior in the light of this question: Are your relationships with old people characterized by sentimentality, or are they—if they exist at all—equal status relationships? Equal status relationships are the key to the kind of treatment that rejects sentimentality and patronizing, that destroys stereotyping and discrimination. Unless we begin to think of old people in terms of individual strengths and skills, individual attractiveness and interest, they will continue a devalued and deprived population, as have other groups in our society, for far longer than is conscionable.

The following exercises should help you begin to cut through the screen of sentimentality and look more objectively at your pattern of interaction with old people.

It helps the process of developing awareness to work on these exercises together with several people, stopping after completing each form individually to express feelings, share observations, and derive strength and comfort from realizing that, although our culture has marked each of us with its debilities, we are still able to question our values and behaviors and, if we wish to do so, to change the quality of our lives.

Exercise A: Identifying People in Your Life

The immediate objective of this exercise is to identify the people you know and categorize them on the basis of level of relationship, from casual acquaintance to intimate friend. Sometimes, it is easy to believe that relationships with certain individuals are closer than they actually are, until we look at them carefully and somewhat analytically. However, before we can probe each relationship, we must begin where we are perceptually—that is, just what do you think your relationships are like?

Before you start to fill in Form 2, make a brief pre-exercise statement on Form 1:

Form 1

On a scale of 1 to 15, how would you rate yourself on your personal involvement with old people? (1 is the lowest, most casual, level of involvement; 15 represents very intimate, personal, equal status involvement, the kind you have with your personal friends.)

Fill in a bar from the base line (labeled Pre-assessment of Relationship with Old People) at 1 to the level at which you think you interact. Save this bar graph for use after you have completed the rest of these exercises.

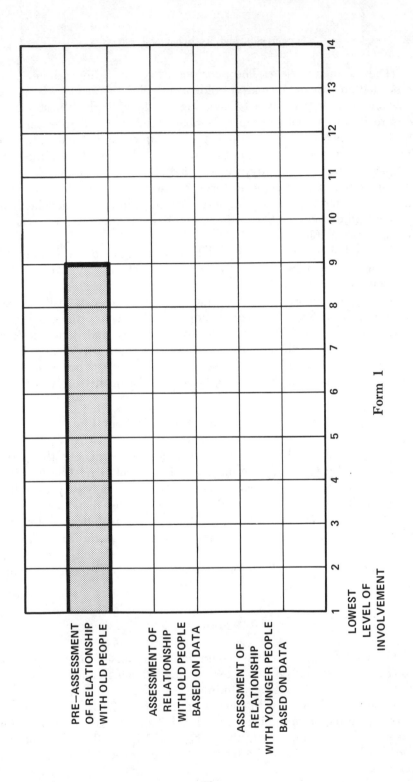

Form 1

Form 2

Follow the directions in the headings of this form, listing the names of the people with whom you interact at different levels.

Level of relationship	List names of people of your age, and up to ten years older or younger.	√	List names of people of your age, and from ten to twenty years older or younger.	√	List names of people under 65 and not yet listed.	√	List names of people over 65.	√
	Make a check mark next to the name of each person who is a close relative of a friend or related to you by blood, marriage, or adoption.						
casual acquaintance							
acquaintance with regular contact							
co-worker (paid or volunteer)							
friend							
good friend							
intimate friend							

In looking at the completed Form 2, do you find a *pattern* of relationships? Does the number of names diminish markedly from level to level of relationship in all the columns? Do you find that there are fewer names at each level as you go from the left-hand column to the right-hand column? Is there a level in a column—or columns—where there are no names at all? Is there a whole column—or columns—where there are no names at all? Are all your friends among the older people related to you in some way?

Does any of this surprise you? How do you explain the pattern?

Exercise B: Analyzing the Levels of Relationship

The objective of this exercise is to identify the behaviors that characterize a particular level of relationship and then to determine if, for example, the word "friend" is applied to young people in exactly the same way it is applied to old people.

Form 3

Take all the names you listed in the columns on Form 2 as friend, good friend, and intimate friend. Under each name, check the activities you regularly engage in with that person. (By regularly, we mean more than once a year or just on special occasions. Use your judgment, but we should think once a month or more often would not be unreasonable for the kinds of activities listed.)

Form 3	30 and younger		50 and younger		65 and younger		over 65	
Activity	name(s)		name(s)		name(s)		name(s)	
1. he (she) confides intimate happenings								
2. have drinks out								
3. meet at parties or informal get-togethers at home of mutual friend								
4. invite to parties or informal gatherings at your home								
5. play cards at home of mutual friend								
6. bike riding								
7. go bowling								
8. he (she) calls you on phone just to chat								
9. call him (her) on phone just to chat								

Activity	30 and younger name(s)					50 and younger name(s)					65 and younger name(s)					over 65 name(s)				
10. share readings—magazines, books, etc.																				
11. plan future activities																				
12. take vacations together																				
13. talk about hair and clothes fashions																				
14. watch TV																				
15. you confide intimate happenings																				
16. go to dinner at his (her) home																				
17. invite to dinner at your home																				
18. go to lunch at her (his) home																				

Activity	30 and younger *name(s)*			50 and younger *name(s)*			65 and younger *name(s)*			over 65 *name(s)*		
19. invite to lunch at your home												
20. have dinner out												
21. go to theater												
22. go to classical concerts												
23. go to rock concerts												
24. go to movies												
25. have lunch out												
26. go to coffee house												
27. go shopping												
28. go out with mutual friends												

Form 4

Now, add the total number of check marks in each age category and plot the numbers on a bar graph. (On page 87 is one student's graph.)

Compare the size of the bar for each age span. Do you see something that interests or surprises you in the comparison? How do you explain the differences? Are you dismayed, or do you feel that your pattern of inter-relationships is perfectly natural?

Exercise C: Examining Relationships with Old People Who Are Relatives or Relatives of Friends

Form 5a

The immediate objective of this exercise is to determine the nature of the relationships with old people who are related beyond just friend-ship. Sometimes, activities that appear to be similar to friendship activi-ties are actually differentially motivated—and even different in quality from friendship behavior.

From Form 2, take all the names that have a check mark next to them indicating an element of consanguinity in the relationship. Insert the names on Form 5a on the designated lines. For each activity engaged in with that person (as indicated on Form 3) check off the reason for it under each person's name. (Some activities will, of course, have more than one check mark.)

For each person listed, add up the total number of checks. Then, for each person, add up only the number of checks next to the activities with asterisks. (The behaviors with asterisks are friendship behaviors.)

Compute the percentage of reasons and qualities that are character-istic of friendship behavior. This is the proportion of friendship behaviors in your total relationship with that person. (The number of checks with asterisks divided by the total number of checks, multiplied by 100.)

Now go back to Form 1 and add a bar that illustrates the answer to this question: On a scale of 1 to 15, how would you rate yourself on your personal involvement with old people? (Remember, 1 is the lowest, most casual level; 15 is very intimate, equal status involvement.)

How do the two bars on Form 1 compare? Have you changed your mind about the nature of your friendship with old people?

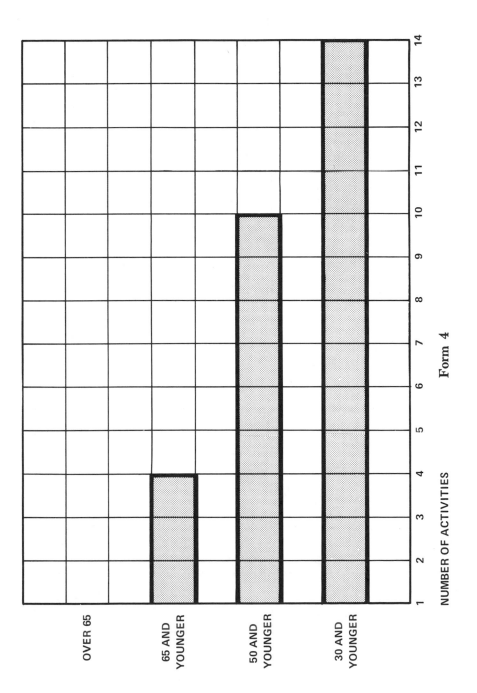

NUMBER OF ACTIVITIES

Form 4

OVER 65

65 AND YOUNGER

50 AND YOUNGER

30 AND YOUNGER

Form 5a

	Name	Name	Name	Name	Name	Name
I'm grateful to her/him						
She was important to me when I was a child						
He/she is an important part of my life °						
She/he needs the exercise						
He/she doesn't get out much						
She/he can't get there without help						
He/she has no one else to go with						
I want to make her/him feel a part of things						
She/he used to be good at it						
He/she gets lonely						
I feel sorry for him/her						
I like being seen with him/her °						
He/she gives me a good game °						
She/he can hold his liquor °						
She/he is a lot of fun °						
I feel guilty if I don't						
She/he knows how to have a good time °						
She/he is a good cook						

	Name	Name	Name	Name	Name	Name
I love him/her *						
We enjoy each other's company *						
He/she doesn't preach *						
I'm proud of my skill *						
He/she has good ideas *						
She/he empathizes *						
He/she has good taste *						
We like the same things *						
He/she keeps asking me to						
We share many similar interests *						
She/he enjoys it						
He/she pays my way						

Exercise D: Examining Relationships with Old People Who Are Not Related

Form 5b

Now take the names of the people in the last column of Form 2 whose names do not appear on Form 5a and repeat the process here, checking off the reasons for various activities with them and computing the percentage of reasons that indicate peer-status friendship.

If there were no names left in the last column of Form 2, what does that tell you about your associations with old people? (For example, the chances are that all your *young* friends are not related to you.)

If you have been able to use Form 5b, can you conclude that you really do have friends who are old?

Form 5b

	Name	Name	Name	Name	Name	Name
I'm grateful to her/him						
She was important to me when I was a child						
He/she is an important part of my life °						
She/he needs the exercise						
He/she doesn't get out much						
She/he can't get there without help						
He/she has no one else to go with						
I want to make her/him feel a part of things						
She/he used to be good at it						
He/she gets lonely						
I feel sorry for him/her						
I like being seen with him/her °						
He/she gives me a good game °						
She/he can hold his liquor °						
She/he is a lot of fun °						
I feel guilty if I don't						
She/he knows how to have a good time °						
She/he is a good cook						

	Name	Name	Name	Name	Name	Name
I love him/her *						
We enjoy each other's company *						
He/she doesn't preach *						
I'm proud of my skill *						
He/she has good ideas *						
She/he empathizes *						
He/she has good taste *						
We like the same things *						
He/she keeps asking me to						
We share many similar interests *						
She/he enjoys it						
He/she pays my way						

Exercise E: Examining Relationships with Young People

Form 5c

Now you might fill in this form as you did Form 5a using the names of your young friends, and compute the percentage of your total activities with each one representing peer-status relationship. How does this figure compare with your results in 5a and 5b?

Form 5c

	Name	Name	Name	Name	Name	Name
I'm grateful to her/him						
She was important to me when I was a child						
He/she is an important part of my life °						
She/he needs the exercise						
He/she doesn't get out much						
She/he can't get there without help						
He/she has no one else to go with						
I want to make her/him feel a part of things						
She/he used to be good at it						
He/she gets lonely						
I feel sorry for him/her						
I like being seen with him/her °						
He/she gives me a good game °						
She/he can hold his liquor °						
She/he is a lot of fun °						
I feel guilty if I don't						
She/he knows how to have a good time °						
She/he is a good cook						

	Name	Name	Name	Name	Name	Name
I love him/her *						
We enjoy each other's company *						
He/she doesn't preach *						
I'm proud of my skill *						
He/she has good ideas *						
She/he empathizes *						
He/she has good taste *						
We like the same things *						
He/she keeps asking me to						
We share many similar interests *						
She/he enjoys it						
He/she pays my way						

Form 1

Now add a bar to the graph (Form 1), representing an assessment of your relationship with younger people. Your completed Form 1 may look like the graph on page 94, which is based on the exercise results of a 23-year-old nursing student in a baccalaureate program.

Discussion of Exercises A–E

You have heard the remark made by some white people, "Some of my best friends are Negroes." Although most of us are aware enough that this testament to tolerance is a thin mask for prejudice, the defense of self continues to crop up in more subtle ways: "I have friends of all races," "It doesn't matter to me what color a person is—black, white, yellow, or green." Such statements are viewed by those who are sensitive to the evidences of prejudice in our culture with considerable scepticism.

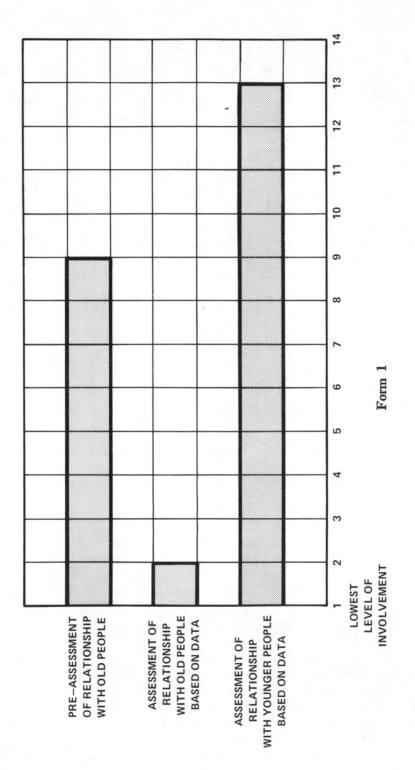

Form 1

At the very least, they question the speaker's definition of friendship as it is applied to Black people. A mild question or two soon makes it clear that this white person's Black "friends" are never invited to her home, she has never visited their homes, and it is unlikely that they have ever done anything together outside of work or school, where they have been compelled to "associate" because of antidiscrimination laws.

Therefore, although at the outset of any program to raise consciousness and reduce discrimination, participants are apt to overestimate their self-assessment concerning cross-race association, by the time the program is over they are usually revising the assessment downward. The less sophisticated often maintain that this growing awareness that they are prejudiced really means that *the program* is *causing* them to be prejudiced, and this can be an uncomfortable period for instructor and students. But reassurance that such self-awareness is evidence of increasing wisdom, and continued perseverance in exploring the realities of intergroup relations, combine to help all participants go on with their deliberations.

As we begin to break down the category of people we call "friends," in our eagerness to prove that we do not indulge in anything so odious as discrimination, we are compelled to admit that not all the people to whom we are *friendly* can honestly be identified as our friends. Even a long-term working relationship, during which we sometimes even have lunch with an older person, cannot be labeled a friendship when we compare it to our relationships with other people in our lives.

However, even when we first begin the analysis (Form 2), it probably begins to become apparent that, even with the most liberal definition of friendship, the largest number of people we call friends are those closest to our own age.

Form 3 begins to pinpoint the nature of these relationships we call friendships. There are generally recognizable activities we engage in with our friends, and we try here to see if these activities are spread across the spectrum of age or limited to those closest to us in years.

In working with people in their twenties and thirties, it is at this point in the exercises that they begin to face the fact that they have not had old or older people as friends, and they slowly begin to examine the reasons that they bring out from deep inside their consciousness. It is here that it becomes clear that a large part of the separation of the age groups is a function of stereotypic thinking.

One idea that keeps coming up—albeit reluctantly—is the fear that friendship with an old person inevitably must be a helping relationship, with the young party to the friendship called upon to assume responsibilities for shopping, chauffeuring, and sick-bed attendance. That this fear is largely unwarranted is revealed by some of the data in the field:

"Rather than being a major segment of the aged, those seriously handicapped by poor health are a small minority. . . . [T]he bulk of the aged actually manage to function quite adequately." [2] However, the professionals in the field continue to contribute to the stereotype of the aged as generally severely impaired: [3]

> Problems of old age are of two general kinds: those that older people actually have and those that experts think they have. This distinction is not simply whimsical, for while the two may overlap, they certainly do not correspond. The difference between them reflects several factors. The old age field attracts many dedicated practitioners who work directly with the aged and, on their behalf, are deeply committed to social action and reform. Indeed, they regard gerontology almost as an ideological movement. Their intense involvement commonly magnifies older people's problems which then seem to loom larger than life and crowd most other issues from their perspective. In the process, their perception is often warped.

Rosow goes on to maintain that ". . . the most significant problems of older people . . . are intrinsically social. The basic issue is that of their social integration." [4] One bar to such integration is the sheer inertia of the status quo. A number of high school students, when the idea was proposed to them, said they had never thought of a friendship relation with an old person; it simply had never occurred to them. When a college student described to them his own experience with the Gray Panthers and the one special friend he had made, they were intrigued with the idea. Upon reflection, they thought they *could* be real friends with an old person. Several of them made a commitment to try to make such a change in their pattern of relationships.

Others engaged the college student in the kind of dialogue exemplified by Allport's classic interchange [5]:

MR. X: The trouble with Jews is that they only take care of their own group.

MR. Y: But the record of the Community Chest campaign shows that they give more generously, in proportion to their numbers, to the general charities of the community, than do non-Jews.

MR. X: That shows they are always trying to buy favor and intrude into Christian affairs. They think of nothing but money; that is why there are so many Jewish bankers.

MR. Y: But a recent study shows that the percentage of Jews in the banking business is negligible, far smaller than the percentage of non-Jews.

Mr. X: That's just it; they don't go in for respectable business; they are only in the movie business or run night clubs.

The dialogue about old people went something like this:

High School Student: You can't have an old person as a friend. All they ever talk about are their aches and pains.

College Student: But the Gray Panthers is an organization of mostly old people who are interested and active in politics and social change.

High School Student: That shows they'd rather associate with their own age group. They formed their own organization instead of participating the way other people do.

College Student: But studies show that old people vote more regularly than many young people do, and are more concerned about political issues.

High School Student: Sure, they want to bring us back to "the good old days"; they don't like change.

College Student: The evidence we have is that old people are not particularly conservative politically. And look at all the young people involved in the nostalgia craze for things of the '50s and '60s.

High School Student: They're still the ones who stand in the way of progress, when they hold on to their jobs and don't give young people a chance to move up.

Both conversations demonstrate the difficulty a person may have in using information that denies the validity of what he believes to be true. It is a testament to the inescapable fact that merely exposing prejudiced people to "the facts" is insufficient to change their way of thinking. The stereotypes that young people hold even seem to be "remarkably resistant to change from exposure to, familiarity and contact with older persons." [6] In reviewing the work in this area, however, I would suggest that the missing intervening variable between contact and reduction of prejudice is the kind of sustained consciousness raising and self-analysis that we are trying to do here.

One often heard reason for avoiding cross-age friendships is an appeal to the "logic" of the situation. After all, young unmarried people are engaged in the natural quest for mates; surely there would be no point in including old people in the activities and concerns leading to success in this quest. The argument collapses when we see young people maintaining friendships even after some of them are married.

In Form 5a we look at the nature of the bond with old people who are close to us, trying to determine if the closeness is based on the need for friendship or on considerations that may even result in destructive relationships. In one discussion of this form, a young nurse told about visiting with her grandmother regularly and how coldly and perfunctorily she performed this duty, and how she suffered from anxiety about what to say and how to respond. Not only did she think it inconceivable that she could ever be friends with an old person, but some of this anxiety was inevitably evoked whenever she came into professional contact with someone old.

Another nurse in the group, who thought that she and her grandfather were "good friends," began to identify in her relationship with him a pattern that required all the giving to be on her side and all the receiving on his. She finally said that the only good she derived from the "friendship" was the satisfaction that she was doing what had to be done. There was no friendship here, and she began to wonder if her grandfather saw this, and, if he did, how it made him feel.

If you believe that old people are truly numbered among your friends (or, if you are old, you number young people among your friends), then your behavior with them should be no different from your behavior with your other friends.

Why do we immediately call small children by their first names, when we insist that they call us by our title and last names? Can it be that we don't see ourselves as our children's equals? Well, can the same thing be said of the difference in address when we interact with old people? How real is a "friendship" between people who are not equals, if the relationship contains elements of subservience, condescension, feelings of superiority?

Friends need to be open with each other, easy with each other. If there is a formality between them, then the formality is reciprocal rather than one-sided, and it is usually a function of the newness of the relationship. Such formality cannot persist among people who begin to engage in their leisure-time activities in each other's company. If you must speak differently to a person because he is older, then you will not be comfortable bowling or jogging with him. You may manage it for a while, but it takes some of the fun out of it if you cannot relax and be yourself.

That term "respect" is used, consciously or unconsciously, to maintain a distance between the older and the younger. The attitude and the behavior it purports to describe is not really respectful: it merely implies, "There are some things I feel that I may not express to you; there are some ways I like to act that I may not in your presence—not because you are wiser or more accomplished, but because you are different from me."

Similarly with this push for protecting the aged. Our equals need no special protection; they have rights and responsibilities as we do, and they are entitled to the same protection that the law provides for us all. I can't help thinking of what happened to children that we wanted to "protect": We arranged it so that they were deprived of almost all the protection of the law that adults got as their right, and juvenile trials became little more than star chamber proceedings in which arbitrary disposition was made of defendants who had no counsel and no opportunity to challenge their accusers.

Now that the Supreme Court has ruled that we must stop "protecting" children and that they must have equal treatment before the law, they may no longer be imprisoned for behavior that is not considered actionable when done by adults.

Evaluating Media

The media which continually bombard us often send out messages that perpetuate error and falsehood. Often, however, the messages are so familiar and are sent to us so frequently that we absorb them automatically, without even being aware of how they influence our thinking and behavior. Consciousness raising about any area of injustice requires a deliberate campaign of noticing what is being done and said, and identifying the errors and lies in the morass of words and deeds.

One of the results of such a personal campaign is to develop such heightened sensitivity that the stereotypes and injustices seem to leap out at us from everywhere—from newspapers and magazines, best-sellers and movies, political speeches and casual conversations. Sometimes, we may even be accused of seeing prejudice where none exists, but this is the price we pay for waking up: those who are still asleep may become impatient with us and the noise we are making. But such sensitivity is an indispensable part of the process of eliminating prejudice, whether it is prejudice between racial groups, between the sexes, or between age groups: If you see no evidence of the problem, you would hardly be motivated to solve it!

You might start with any daily newspaper. Read it from first page to last, looking for evidences of the state of relationships with old people in the local community, in the state, the nation, and the world. Examine the headlines, the news articles, the columns, the editorials, the picture advertisements, and the classified sections. Read the sports pages and the advice to the lovelorn. Read the comic strips and the cartoons.

Each time you come to an item that reveals something about attitudes toward old people, make a note of it. If you are doing this in a group, call out each time you find something and share it with the others.

Here are some examples found in a big city newspaper on one day together with a comment or two on their significance:

On Friday, July 2, 1976, the *Philadelphia Daily News* [7] wrote about the traditions on which America is built. (The nostalgia for the past is, of course, a part of the July 4 celebration, especially in the bicentennial year.) However, none of the allusions to tradition included an appreciation of the old, who, presumably, are tradition-bound.

There *was* an account of a music festival [8] in which none of the performers were identified by age except "Eubie Blake: 93-year-old master," who was pictured in the article with this caption. His age was repeated again in the story, and his music evaluated also in terms of his age: ". . . he makes virtuoso use of his advanced age to get certain universal truths across." I cannot really understand what this means, but it sounds suspiciously like a rhetorical vehicle for emphasizing the man's age. Lurking in the background is the echo of a fatuous: "Isn't it wonderful! At his age!"

In the amusements and book section [9] an unnamed writer mentioned "My retired friend from Maine . . ." who did not like a book. Here, again, it is not clear why the descriptive "retired" was necessary in this allusion. It sounds almost like "My Black friend read this mystery story. . . ." What can it matter that the friend was Black if the story had nothing in it that needed the special interpretation of someone who has had the Black experience in America? It is the sort of thing people do who are still uncomfortable about race, and are trying to prove that they are not.

A letter from a reader [10] takes issues with another reader who apparently has objected to the reduced fare for "senior citizens" on the public transportation. She identifies the recipients of this benefit as among "the most needy of society" and suggests: "Maybe their riding on buses all day is the only enjoyable outing they have access to—at least it's the only type they can afford." Then she warns: "Wait until you get old, living off Social Security and possibly a pension, and you can't afford a car to take you where you want to go."

In this one brief letter, we get a significant portion of the picture of the old held by people in this city. Although many people of all ages use the public transportation—generally for the purposes of getting from one place to the other—there are old people who ride just as a pastime. The questions: Can they enjoy nothing else because they cannot *afford* other activities, or are there no activities that are suitable for them in the city? Maybe what they need more than reduced fares are reduced admissions to movies, theaters, and museums? But then, why is their problem different from the problem of poor people of any age? Do we really have an age problem in this society, or do we have a poverty problem?

The questions call to mind Irving Rosow's observations: "The critical issue is that health problems have financial as well as medical implications" [11] and "The aged simply do not need special housing so much as decent ordinary housing at a price they can afford." [12] And Kent's categorical "Much research indicates that the best prophylactic against a miserable old age is 'to be rich.'" [13]

A real estate columnist gives advice about capital gains exemption for selling one's home after age 65, making it clear that the seller had better seek legal advice before he tries it because the Internal Revenue Service gives conflicting information. [14] And a financial columnist maintains that there is "something almost obscene about a law that permits payment of full Social Security benefits to the wealthy resident of an apartment hotel, living on a generous corporation pension and income from stocks and bonds, while slashing or wiping out the benefits of the chambermaid "because she is working." [15]

In both cases, the essential problem would seem to be money, with age only an incidental factor. That is, although the tax exemption and the Social Security benefit are given to old people, the problem of the beneficiaries is not so much age as it is an inequitable distribution of financial advantages. The articles say something about the official unfairness and, perhaps, a growing awareness of it.

The final item that caught my eye was a number of interviews with people in the street. [16] Three of the four people interviewed were identified by their full names, and under the picture of each was his last name. The fourth person was called Charlie in the interview and under his photograph. He was 84 years old and retired.

In going through this issue of the newspaper, it was easy to see that advertising models were not old, classified job ads did not ask for old people, the columnists pictured did not appear to be old, and the activities reported on all seemed to deal with people who were not old. This in a city where some 11.7 percent of the population is over the age of 65.

Clarifying Values

Now that you have explored the problem of ambivalence and pinpointed the tendency to stereotype, decide what you would do in specific situations when you are faced with a choice of responses. Ask yourself what criteria you use in responding to the circumstances. Are you consistent in your reasoning and logic, or do your various responses betray your own conflicts? Are you more or less comfortable in the different situations? Is the level of comfort always a function of the age of the person in the situation? How do you adjust your behavior so as to increase your comfort? Do you avoid responding at all? Is age a factor in your response only when the person is related to you? Only when he is not related to you?

Each one of the item—or the whole list—can be used as a basis for discussion. During such discussion, no one should be forced to reveal his responses. Individuals might prefer to continue to think about their responses privately. It is possible that, pinned down to the necessity for predicting an attitude in a specific situation, they discover that they simply need more time to examine their own attitudes before they come to a decision, and this need should be respected.

What would you do if

1. She came to you and said she was contemplating marriage?
   Your 21-year-old niece _____
   Your 71-year-old grandmother _____

2. He told you he wanted to become a nurse?
   Your 21-year-old nephew _____
   Your 60-year-old uncle _____

3. He said he wanted to learn how to bowl?
   Your 18-year-old cousin _____
   Your 80-year-old father _____

4. He said he was joining an art class?
   Your 16-year-old brother _____
   Your 73-year-old grandfather _____

5. She was planning to campaign actively for a presidential candidate?
   Your 22-year-old niece _____
   Your 75-year-old patient _____

6. She was going to start college after being out of school for years?
   Your 30-year-old aunt _____
   Your 60-year-old aunt _____

7. He wanted to learn a trade?
   Your 20-year-old patient _____
   Your 65-year-old patient _____

8. She started coming home at two and three in the morning?
   Your 21-year-old sister _____
   Your 70-year-old grandmother _____

9. He became an old-movie buff and started to travel around to see old movies wherever they were shown?
   Your 16-year-old brother _____
   Your 65-year-old grandfather _____

10. All he ever did for recreation was play cards?
    Your 25-year-old cousin _____
    Your 70-year-old uncle _____

Notes

1. This section is adapted from my book, *Affective Subjects in the Classroom: Exploring Race, Sex and Drugs,* Intext Educational Publishers, New York, 1972, pp. 93–106.

2. Irving Rosow, *Social Integration of the Aged,* The Free Press, New York, 1957, p. 3.

3. Ibid., p. 1.

4. Ibid., p. 8.

5. Gordon W. Allport, *The Nature of Prejudice,* Addison-Wesley Publishing Company, Inc., Reading, Mass., 1954, pp. 13–14.

6. Rosow, op. cit., p. 32.

7. *Philadelphia Daily News,* July 2, 1976.

8. Ibid., p. 34.

9. Ibid., p. 29.

10. Ibid., p. 23.

11. Rosow, op. cit., p. 4.

12. Ibid., p. 7.

13. Kent, op. cit.

14. *Philadelphia Daily News,* op. cit., p. 66.

15. Ibid., p. 16.

16. Ibid., p. 10.

attitudes
and behaviors
of professionals

The Professional Perspective

"Social workers are themselves victims of the myths and stigmas associated with the elderly." [1]

". . . in nursing, both collegiate and hospital schools have had little content in geriatric nursing until very recently." [2]

"A review of the catalogues of the academic year 1969–1970 from 99 medical schools revealed that instruction in gerontological subjects was fragmentary or non-existent. . . . This marginal attention from medical institutions probably stems, in large part, from the negative attitude of medical students and practitioners, as far as gerontological subjects are concerned." [3]

". . . our society acculturates dependency and . . . much of the talk about being independent is just so much window dressing. Many gerontologists . . . are busily fostering dependence while loudly proclaiming that they are maintaining independence." [4]

"At the beginning of the course at Catholic University for nurses, social workers and students in other fields, the majority of the students were not free from the common prejudices held by members of this society concerning the aged." [5]

Given these findings, it is not surprising that professionals engaged in the care of the aged are too often insensitive to their needs. Take the case of the old man who speaks hesitantly because he knows that his memory has been affected and he is reluctant to reveal his debility. He speaks in a very low voice, and slowly. His physician, a well-known geriatric specialist, sees him every five or six months for a rather superficial examination.

In the course of the examination, he will ask, in a voice unnecessarily loud, "How are you feeling?" *He never waits long enough for the old man to respond.* After two seconds, he will turn to the man's paid companion and ask—in a more normal voice—"How does he feel?" The patient is left in even greater self-doubt, more disheartened than ever, since it has been made clear that he no longer has the ability to communicate effectively.

"Do you exercise?" the great man shouts. "Do you walk every day?" And before the old man—*who is not hard of hearing*—can begin to relate what he does, the doctor is already giving instructions to "get dressed and come into the office when you're ready." The questions are obviously just perfunctory, since he gets little or no information when he asks them.

One woman whose 70-year-old father lives with her experienced this kind of examination recently. The physician shouted at her father (who *also* is not deaf), "You must keep busy! Do you do something every day?" Although he didn't wait for an answer, the question echoed in her head long after they had left the office. Her father must "do something" every day. She racked her brain to devise activities for him, cutting short her working day so she could take him to a park, to a museum, to a matinee. She hired a man to take him swimming several times a week, to take him to a social center to play bridge. Life for her and her father became a whirl of activity, in an attempt to follow the doctor's casual prescription.

Through it all, she was faced with daily resistance from her father. He reacted to each new activity with, at best, reluctance, and, at worst, with outright distaste. He didn't want to go swimming in the winter, even if the pool was an indoor one and heated. He didn't want to play bridge with strangers—he just didn't want to play cards. Why did he have to go to the museum? He preferred to sit and watch television.

His daughter teased and cajoled him into compliance. When he flatly refused to do something, she burst into anger, partly because she was tired, and partly because she was afraid that if she relaxed the pressure, her father's health would be irreversibly damaged.

One day, when she was spilling over to a friend about how tired with all this activity planning she was, how she was at her wits' end trying to get her father to go along with *her* plans, how an acquaintance had observed only last night that the most important thing is to keep the old person involved and active, her friend asked, "What sort of things did he like to do when he was younger?"

The off-hand question hit her with all the force of a purely original idea. It shook her into sanity and started her remembering her father's life after he had retired from work at the age of 60. For ten years he had lived alone, apparently quite content with his life. He cooked an occasional meal for himself, but mostly he ate in a small family restaurant in the neighborhood. He went to a movie once a week or so. He sat in the park reading a newspaper every day. He rarely engaged in conversation with other people around him—he had never been a gregarious man. He had no hobbies, no special interests. Once his work was over, he had no special thing he liked to do. That was the pattern of his life. Except for his work—that had *always* been the pattern of his life.

Now, just because a physician (who did not know him and was too busy and too indifferent to take the trouble to know him) said he was to do something every day, she was insanely trying to impose a completely new style of life on him. He was being told that life begins at seventy— and begins in a totally new way, as if his personality, his likes, and his dislikes no longer defined him. Life begins at seventy as a different person!

Obviously, from what we have learned about attitudes in our society, this kind of insensitivity cannot be understood *merely* in terms of ignorance, or inability to empathize, or just ordinary distraction because of a busy schedule. I really believe that the primitive approach to intergroup relations is the modus operandi in our culture. For example, although we like to think that we are a child-centered society, actually adult relationships with children are characterized by distrust and punitiveness. I do not refer to those isolated cases of adults who severely beat and even kill their children; I am talking about the vast majority of normal adults, most of whom are parents, and some of whom have had professional training in the care and education of children. Among teachers, the distrust and hostility directed against children is rationalized as a need to maintain control in the classroom. Student teachers are warned not to smile until Christmas; presumably by then the children will have learned to submit to teacher domination, and a smile will not be interpreted as an invitation to disruption.

Parents generally keep an eye out for what children do wrong and are quick to punish "for their own good." In the process of growing up, what children do *right* is seldom deemed worthy of mention—except, perhaps, to strangers.

The truth is that much of the way we deal with children is punitive and destructive. We exclude them from school if they show initiative and independence or are overwhelmed by problems that no one is helping them solve. We label them stupid if they cannot speak English, or incorrigible if they resist the demands to learn irrelevant trivia. We remand them to institutions where they get no schooling and where they are sexually and otherwise assaulted by adults. If they have handicaps, no educational provision is made for them, even though the law has recently been reinterpreted to guarantee them an education. If they run away from intolerable conditions, we call them delinquent. If they murder someone, we say they have committed an "adult" crime and so are not deserving of consideration as children.

Since children are, in essence, a captive population, completely subject to the will of adults, there is an analogy to be made between their condition and the condition of old people who have been forced to trade their independence for sustenance. And it is essentially the same population of adults that dominates these older adults. The similarities of adult attitudes and behavior toward children and old people merit some consideration.

Just as we insert each child into a small space in a vast organization called a school system, and proceed to program him without much regard for his essential individuality, so are we speaking of providing mass care for old people. So much a part of our culture has mass-produced education become that we are usually outraged at any suggestion that our organization of schooling is not a good thing. Now our organization of provisions for the aged in "Senior Citizens' Centers" and "Golden Age Communities" and special housing developments and "Homes" is taking on many of the aspects of assembly-line schooling.

Children who are ridden by anxieties concerning race and sex and drugs are forbidden to air their feelings or deal systematically with their problems in school. Instead, they are forced to spend their time accepting from their teachers bits of unconnected information and giving back these bits on tests. This is the basic idiocy of the schools.

The analogous idiocy in nursing homes, where people live because they have no place else to go, is the almost universal proscription against sex and alcohol. Adults who have lived the ordinary, normal lives that characterize our culture, and have become accustomed to drinking and having sexual relations, are suddenly told that they may not continue to live their normal lives. Why? Because the people who run the home have decided that they may not.

Children are sent to their schooling segregated from any adults with whom they might develop easy, friendly relationships. The only adults with whom they come into contact are those who rule them.

Similarly, the push for provision of adequate housing for old people is concerned not only with physical adaptations for infirmities, but it becomes clear that the housing will be separated from other housing, and old people will be isolated from children and from younger adults—except those who rule them: the housing manager and maintenance people, medical personnel, and social workers.

One can be sure that failure to conform to the rules laid down will be viewed as undesirable. There may even be the implied threat of some punitive action if conformity is resisted. If children in a detention facility (a large number of whom are not criminals but merely neglected or abandoned or have stayed out of school) are denied food for infraction of the rules, how far is it to the denial of food to old people for infraction of the rules? The *power* to do this is often the operative factor in establishing this behavior.

Clues to the national propensity for the systematic destruction of groups that have no power surround us. Look at how we support each other in our need to absolve ourselves of responsibility for our aged parents.

Recently, I heard a physician being interviewed by a TV commentator on the subject of senility. He described the symptoms of some of the degenerative diseases of old age, talking about inability to remember recent events, difficulties in concentration, motor debilities, and so on. He described the old person who asks the same question over and over again, forgetting each time that he has asked it, and forgetting too that he has heard the answer. He also told about people who cannot tie their shoe-laces, or dress themselves, or bathe, or go to the toilet by themselves. He mused aloud about how frustrating it must be to be inside a body that no longer will do one's bidding, so that what you have been accustomed to doing all your life is no longer possible. And he talked about how impatient relatives become when they have to repeat the same things over and over again, or leave their own pursuits to care for the old person.

Then, with a leap that defied all logic of sequence, the interviewer asked, "So many people I talk to feel so guilty about putting their parents or grandparents into homes when this happens. Isn't it really better for them?" (The absence of logic lies in the assumption that there is an inevitable sequence from the beginning of failing faculties to relegation to an institution. There was no talk at all about how to manage a reasonably comfortable life when one member of the family is having such difficulties. On the contrary, the whole process of degenerative disease was labeled senility, and the person who was beginning to fail was called senile. What can one do with the senile but put them away?)

In answer to the interviewer's question, the doctor said sympathetically,

> Every person who is young today will have to face this problem. There's no avoiding it. The thing to remember is that every living thing has its day. Like the flower. It's spring now, and you can enjoy the flowers. But fall will come, and the flowers will be finished. Life will go on because the flower lived.
>
> You must consider where the old person will be more comfortable. And he'll be more comfortable where he can be taken care of.
>
> Now sometimes, if they are aware of what is happening to them, they still won't understand. They'll ask, "What is it? Don't you love me any more? Why don't you love me any more?" But putting them in a home doesn't mean you don't love them. You still love them, so it's not necessary to feel guilty.

The week preceding this interview, a program on the same station had detailed the horrors of old peoples' homes. It showed old people lying for days in their own wastes. There were places that drugged the old into mindless passivity so that no one would be bothered by their complaints, or by their wanting to walk when the staff wanted them to sit. Some old people were literally starved by the unbalanced meals. Others were tied to their beds "for their own good."

Finally, the program had closed with the homily that has been used as a disclaimer ever since the situation in nursing homes came to light: Of course, not *all* homes for the aged are bad. *Some* are very good.

There seems to be some difficulty in determining exactly what "good" means in this context, since institutional care is apparently enormously expensive, and neither government nor most private citizens are able to pay adequately for institutional care of old people. Presumably, then, the "good" homes are used by extremely wealthy individuals; I wonder just how many such homes for the aged there are in this country.

There is something else to be considered, too, in the matter of assessing the quality of care in any institution. Institutions foster a process of depersonalization that neither money nor professional skill is able to mitigate. The efficient nurse's reference to "the gallbladder in 240" is an example of how the person is often subsumed to the specific cause of institutionalization, and the gallbladder is treated as if there were not a unique individual attached to it. Such efficiency carried to the ultimate horrible absurdity is the practice of bathing old people on an assembly-line kind of arrangement, with no thought to individual modesty or individual differences in ability to care for one's own personal needs.[6] Here old age is the reason for institutionalization, old age is equated with loss of ability, so people are treated as if they have lost all ability to respond in their unique human ways.

The man who is tied to his bed "for his own good" is not given consideration for being someone who has, for most of his life, made his way to the bathroom in the middle of the night. There is no real attempt to ascertain if he is still able to do this in the institutional setting. The fact that he is old and now finds himself in an unfamiliar place is reason enough to "protect" him by tying him down.

Similarly, the young nurse who *loves* all old people and the middle-aged aide for whom the work is a grinding back-breaking bore both nullify what is human in the people for whom they provide institutional care. The unique individual who, up until this point, has lived his own life in his own way is no longer responded to as if he were unique. It is almost as if he has suddenly become a unit indistinguishable from numbers of other units, the end result of a process of mass production. The care, also, becomes a mass-produced ministration, with everyone getting the same screw tightened, whether he needs it or not.

This whole process requires that strangers be the ministrators. People whom you have nurtured cannot stereotype you. People with whom you have shared a home may dislike you personally, but they cannot deny that you are a unique human being, different from all other human beings. People with whom you share memories cannot believe that your feelings are the same as the feelings of the other people in the institution. Only strangers can believe that all old people want to celebrate Christmas, or prefer to live exclusively with other old people, or are content to watch television all day, or are willing to let others make decisions for them.

The very young and the very old are particularly vulnerable when they are enmeshed in this kind of process. The very young die of a kind of malnutrition of the spirit. The very old do the same. The tensions of living in a familial environment are what nourish people. The conflict, the love, the holding, the hurts, the celebrations are the food of life. The bland, colorless, isolating "efficiency" of an institution lulls one to death.

Given all the information we have about existing institutions, the physician and the interviewer still complacently accepted as unarguable the expectation that the very old need to be institutionalized. And when you have had your day, that will be the best thing for you, too!

The sort of statement that follows is what helps to reinforce in our society the idea that the most viable alternatives for the care of the aged are living alone or, failing that, living in an institution: "Ask almost any old person what it is he really wants in his remaining years, and he will say he wants to be able to take care of himself in his own home or apartment. Unfortunately, large numbers of elderly people in failing physical or mental health are forced to go to institutions. The phenomenon of the nursing home is an increasing one, and the numbers of old people entering such facilities have made the nursing homes a major 'industry' in our culture." [7]

The almost careless skipping of the third possibility—living with one's offspring—shows a selectivity in the perception of researchers that is the result of our general reluctance to accept this alternative. To the extent that we, just as carelessly, accept such a statement without question, to that extent will we continue to contribute to the growth of the nursing home industry, complacent in the belief that the specialists in the field have examined the data and found the solutions. What we overlook is the fact that the specialists in the field are themselves adult offspring of aged parents, and so a prey to the same social and psychological pressures that we all react to.

The fact remains that the overwhelming majority of old people live with their families or in their own homes. If some of the money for government projects for study and care of the old were *given* to the old, both they and their families would be having an easier time of it trying to make ends meet, providing for such mundane and necessary things as taxis to and from doctors' offices, delivery service for groceries, and heavy cleaning and repairing chores. In the long run it would probably cost us less in money, and far, far less in human unhappiness.

I don't care how good nursing homes are—they are no answer to the need we all have for living out our lives with dignity. No institution is. The money poured into those things would be far better used by families to provide a place for aged parents with them. And doctors and social workers would do better to stop the practice of being so quick to encourage families to put their old people into these places—better to help educate sons and daughters to the value of learning to live again with their parents.

As it is, professionals make much of easing the feelings of guilt that offspring have when they cannot accept the challenge and responsibility of providing a home for someone who can no longer live alone. When have they ever performed such a function before? What right have they now to make things easier for the young by making them more difficult for the old?

I think we can concede that most professionals are neither cruel nor uncaring. But it must also be conceded that those who are paid to "care" are only paid lovers. At best they can feel a passing spark of interest, a burst of affection. But when the working day is over, they go home to the families and friends they *really* love. Whatever skill and knowledge they possess, they will provide to their charges and their patients; whatever devotion they have to give will be given to their own.

That is why there can be no substitute plans for caring for the aged. They must have their own families and friends about them who knew and loved them when they were young. The debilities of age are comforted and eased in the company of those who have loved for a lifetime, not those who are being paid to simulate love. If there is to be governmental intervention in the caring of the aged, it should be the kind that provides the wherewithal to help families stay together, not the kind that gives impetus to our baser urges for management, efficiency, and assembly-line organization.

While the impetus to change the attitudes and behavior of Americans toward the old grows stronger, work proliferates apace on designing environments for the aged. "There are facilities for the indigent elderly, apartments built by private operators, retirement communities supported by agencies, institutions for sheltered care, day centers, golden age clubs, and sheltered work opportunities. . . ." [8]

Part of the on-going development involves studies of a variety of psychological and physical factors in an attempt to ascertain the physical surroundings and the psychological atmosphere that would provide optimum conditions for the aged. One statement by such a researcher, admittedly taken out of context of a report of various attempts to amass data for use in making life productive and comfortable for old people, makes one tremble with the intimations for the future with its Orwellian undertones: [9]

A possibility involves establishing environments in which the older person will encounter novel, uncertain, conflicting, and complex stimulations. If we can control these aspects of stimulation, we can discover whether curiosity and activity are increased. In environments in which these attributes are varied, we could measure the activity and the participation of older people by observational methods. We might even be able to maximize novelty while holding uncertainty, conflict and complexity at moderate levels or work out any other combination and then study the outcomes for activity and participation.

In attempting to "reverse the process of disengagement," and in the name of research, old people will be provided playpens that provide optimal stimulation. It is an absurd approach to so many problems in our society that focuses on studying and changing the victim, while the social forces and individuals that perpetuate the victimization are left free—and even encouraged—to continue their ways.

The professionals seem, barely regretfully, resigned to segregation: "Thus the central cities are increasingly becoming the dwelling places of ethnic minorities, and of the elderly of all groups. . . . The other place of concentration for older persons dwelling is the smaller towns in the farm states: the younger families are moving out of these states, while the retirees move from the farm to the nearby village or town. . . . Older people are likely to be increasingly 'segregated' in American society." [10]

This would seem to be the time to abandon the archaic nonjudgmental descriptive studies and devote some time to developing a truly value-laden gerontology. Such a science does not focus on describing old people and experimenting with making changes within the parameters of the status quo; it questions the basic tenets of our society by examining the consequences—in human destruction—of contemporary attitudes and behaviors.

The "vast institutional shrug of the shoulders" [11] in the diagnosis and treatment of the old that I saw in a large general hospital is often replicated in individual professionals—even those who profess to devote their lives to the care of the aged. [12]

[It] is easier for some doctors to attribute the behavior of the aged patient to "incurable" brain damage than to consider all the purely emotional factors or the effect of medications as the cause, especially when our psychiatrists do the same thing all too often.

A recent study by the National Institute of Mental Health indicated that more than half of our psychiatrists *never* deal with aged patients. Those who do, spend less than 4 percent of their available time with them —an average of less than one hour per week devoted to their care of the aged. This is not because the aged patient doesn't have major psychiatric difficulties; it reflects the too-widespread feeling that nothing can be done for such a patient except feed him, keep him clean and comfortable, and await the inevitable end with resignation.

Family members who live with aged parents become the buffers between the unfeeling professional and the old person they are committed to nurture. And the buffers often emerge from the experience bruised and bleeding. There is the experience of one man whose father is 84 years old. They visit the geriatrist regularly for what appear to be superficial examinations—weight, blood pressure, heart, lungs, and palpation here and there. No treatment is needed or given, though the doctor's bill always reads, "Examination, evaluation, and treatment." That, and the date of the visit and the charge, are the only things that appear on the bill.

One day, after the usual visit, the bill that came to the house had on it "Diagnosis: Arteriosclerotic Heart Disease." Never, in the two years of regular visits, had any mention been made of this disease. The old man was apparently in good health, and there had been no visible deterioration of his condition during that time.

The son was very disturbed when he saw the bill, and spent an agonizing few hours wondering how to tell his father that he was apparently suffering from a serious disease. He finally was able to reach the doctor and ask for more information about the diagnosis.

"You never said he had heart disease!" he protested to the doctor.

"Oh, *everybody* over 60 has some arteriosclerosis," he answered impatiently. "There's nothing you have to do about it."

Nothing you have to do about it except lose a night's sleep!

Although waiting in doctors' offices seems to be a national pastime that people have come to accept with some equanimity, it seems to me that doctors with large geriatric practices force the pastime to absurd lengths. The old people sit patiently for two and three and four hours, often unable even to look at a magazine because the light is so dim. But they never seem to complain—and the doctor never seems to apologize to them for keeping them waiting.

Once I sat with my father for *five hours*, in the waiting room of a well-known orthopedist. We had an appointment, and we were there early for it. The doctor had not been called out, and didn't seem to have any unexpected difficulties. Apparently, three and four appointments had been made for each 10-minute time segment, and the people were just expected to wait. (Hairdressers that cater to wealthy women would not *dare* to schedule their appointments in this way. Why is it deemed acceptable when physicians do it? And how often do nurses abet this behavior and justify it?)

When my father and I came in, the seats were all taken, and three old people (one on crutches) were leaning against a wall. I insisted that the receptionist—hidden behind opaque glass—get me a chair from somewhere in the inner recesses of the examining rooms. After some argument, she nastily told me I could come in and get one myself. My father and I shared that chair for five hours, before he was called in, told to undress, and left to sit in one of a row of 3-foot by 3-foot half-curtained cubbyholes for another hour. Each cubbyhole had a person in it, and they reminded me of the cows I had seen in the stalls of a huge dairy, waiting expressionlessly for their turns at the milking machine.

My reaction to this experience was a burning rage that must have corroded the linings of my throat and stomach. I vowed never to go near that doctor again. But the damage to my body and mind had been done. Was the quiet acceptance by all the old people of this outrage another example of what had happened to a group that is without power?

It apparently is not only in this country that the professionals who offer services to the aged are revealing their attitudes. "They make insufficient differentiation between old people," Coleman, quoting Jones, says of Great Britain, "and do not focus resources at the point of need. . . . Further, there is need for more sensitivity in asking old people what they want. Many elderly hesitate to seek help because they have a dread of being organized by the officious middle-aged." [13]

The outmoded idea of "disengagement"—a process that gradually removes the individual from that kind of interaction that has characterized his life up to the point that he has been labeled "old"—seems in many ways to be more than just a professional researcher's description of an observed process. Broad general inferences are made from the basic definition, not only by lay people but by professionals, and old people are defined in terms of these inferences.

For example, it is assumed that if a person is suffering from some kind of ailment, it is to be expected that he will naturally be inclined to "disengage" himself from his usual activities and roles. I cannot help remembering the observation that most of the work of the world is done by people who don't feel very well. It would seem, from even the most casual observation, that disengagement is a fluctuating function of our whole lives, and our involvements increase or decrease in number and intensity as we feel better or worse, physically and mentally. I would suggest, then, that disengagement as a function is *imposed* on the definition of old age, as if it were a process exclusively of old age. Given this definition, old people are, by extension, seen as disengaged. Then we are moved to justify the institutions that hasten the disengagement, even though they may be doing so for reasons that are not justifiable.

An industry may force retirement on all its employees at the age of 65, because actuarial tables indicate that more people over the age of 65 suffer from certain chronic diseases than younger people do. The implication is that the work of the business will not be done by those over 65. But the fact is that the implication is not warranted. There are businesses and institutions that continue effectively (as effectively as *any* business functions!) with a significant number of its employees over the age of 65. And all businesses function with their many *younger* employees suffering from chronic illnesses, during which they continue to work. They may take days off, they may be less efficient one day than another, but they do get the job done. A man of 70 with the same disease would not be given the chance to show that he can get the job done just as well.

But belief in the validity of disengagement after 65 gets added impetus from the manner in which the social security laws are written. Despite the repeated assertion that you can't legislate attitudes (used primarily as an argument against antidiscrimination laws), the fact is that law *can* affect attitudes. There is nothing so powerful in determining the rightness of behavior as being able to say, "It's the law." So the idea of major disengagement at 65 is firmly institutionalized, and with disengagement from work we are primed for disengagement from most other status functions and prestige roles.

Seeming to accept the inevitability of disengagement without question, one student of social gerontology defines old age not only as "the beginning of the end," but he adds: "Loneliness and boredom are thought to be common. This is not apt to be a very pleasant period." [14] Later [15] he suggests that a *symptomatic* approach to defining the stages of later life would be preferable to a chronological approach if there were some satisfactory way of identifying older people symptomatically. He goes on to suggest the factors that might appear in a quantifying scale, and here loneliness and boredom are included as two of the symptoms. This is the way we human beings take the status quo and transform it into an authoritative standard.

It is true that the widespread perception of old people is that they are lonely and bored—more lonely and bored, presumably, than are middle-aged and young people. This may or may not be true of our society. Nor do we know this to be true of other societies. But we seem slowly to be accepting as fact that boredom and loneliness are somehow a natural function of old age, which can be somewhat mitigated but not really dealt with seriously. Thus, instead of providing institutional supports that maintain opportunities for individuals to continue to live their lives in their own way, the thrust of "programing" for the aged is to provide "recreation" or to encourage volunteerism, both of which more often than not complete the individual's deteriorating self-concept. How worthwhile can the person consider himself, in a culture that values the earning of money, when he spends all his days in group games or in doing work for which he is offered no remuneration? At best, the time passes with an appearance of involvement, while the essential loneliness and the self-doubts continue.

How many of those who are pursuing research on aging learn about themselves what one group of data gatherers, social scientists, and psychiatrists did? "Overprotection, too much respect, an exaggerated admiration or politeness which held them at a distance, a conviction that the old were entirely different from themselves, all of these disguises for prejudice had to be recognized and overcome. . . ." [16]

But the physician who made the following observation still has much to learn about himself: [17]

Many old patients are either garrulous or hesitant in their speech. Their memory may be poor, and some are afflicted by an excessively vivid imagination. They often do not understand that the doctor simply cannot make them better through his own skill and initiative, but that they must actively cooperate and strive in every way, every day, to get better and better.

They phone the doctor, asking him to visit them when this is quite unnecessary, and when all they can gain from him is reassurance. These patients consume more than their share of the hard-pressed, overworked physician's time. Since most old folks have depressed incomes, the well-intentioned doctor can wreck his practice by serving as guide, philosopher, and friend to too many geriatric patients.

The Administration on Aging has called for research on "Attitudes Toward The Elderly Among Professionals" that bodes well for the future of professional education. They define the importance of the problem: [18]

A positive or negative attitude on the part of professionals toward the group which they are serving affects the quality of service provided. As an advocate for older persons, the Administration on Aging desires to foster positive attitudes in the professional communities toward older persons. It is important to know what information is available which describes the types of attitudes prevalent among different groups of professionals. This information is necessary to determine what additional research might be needed in this area, and what methods of enhancing positive attitudes might be more successful.

With the advent and rapid proliferation of machines, the service profession continues to be a major source of livelihood for more and more people. Unlike the mechanical single-step functioning required on the assembly line, service work is comfortably justified in humanistic terms. Our American Creed, which implies that people are important, and which is fed to us with our mid-morning snacks in nursery school, provides a values framework that reinforces the economic-industrial trend. So people become nurses, teachers, aides of all kinds—and social workers. Unfortunately, the institutional forms of these professions have a tendency to make the service as unhumanistic as service can be. Some of the consequences of being served may actually cause suffering that might conceivably have been avoided if there were no such system.

Take the case of the 70-year-old woman who became totally blind within a period of three months. She had been living alone for twenty years and managing her life quite well. A daughter who lived several miles away was taken up with her own two small children and visited her mother only occasionally. The old woman, unable to use the public transportation without assistance, had not left her own neighborhood for about five years.

With her rapidly failing sight, she was forced to ask for assistance from the public welfare agency. The agency assigned a case worker who decided that the woman needed a homemaker during the day, someone to do the housework and prepare the meals, help the woman dress, and walk out with her during the day. The daughter was relieved—her mother would be adequately cared for.

Once every two or three weeks the daughter would come to see how her mother was doing. Each time she found the old woman in bed. Each time she was told, "I don't feel very well. I'll just stay in bed until I feel better." The daughter reckoned that her mother was old; she was getting feeble. At least she had someone taking care of her. Everything was under control.

The social worker, after bringing the homemaker the first day, was not able to visit again for two months. She had a heavy case load, and this woman's need had been adequately provided for.

The homemaker left the job after two months, and she was replaced by another one. This woman discovered that the description of her client provided by the case worker was not accurate. The woman apparently never got out of bed. She was almost completely helpless, needing bedpans and unable to move much even to have her bed linens changed. She sat up a little to eat only with great difficulty. The old woman never talked.

This homemaker took it upon herself to inquire about the woman's medical history and discovered that there was no medical reason for her to be bedridden. When she tried to get her out of bed, however, the woman was unable to stand, so weak were her leg muscles from disuse. However, she persevered, until the old woman was able to get about without assistance. In the process of rehabilitating her client, she discovered that the other homemaker had never talked to her. She would come in, slap some tasteless, cold food in front of her, and then go into the living room and watch television. Slowly, the old woman had stopped talking and stopped trying to live normally. It had just been by the purest chance that someone had finally been assigned to her who cared what happened. The social worker and the woman's daughter might not have discovered the true state of affairs for years—if at all. Even the neighbors accepted as "natural" that an old blind woman should finally be forced to take to her bed. Thank heaven the government provided expert help; at least our taxes were spent to *some* good purpose!

The point of the story is that, if expert service workers had not been involved in the situation, the old woman might have had a better chance at continuing her life in comfort. But everyone thought that the people in charge had the situation well in hand. Of course, the point also is that one service worker, who took the objectives of her profession seriously, was instrumental in salvaging a life. Practitioners in the helping professions are certainly needed; they do jobs that must be done—and often with empathy and a high level of competence. However, part of the problem of patients and other service recipients and their families is that they are often ambivalent about asking for help, about admitting a need. In addition, in the drive to be helpful, service professionals may foist on them services that they neither need nor want—especially if their agency does not offer what the person does need. The result is a total experience for patient and family that is abrasive and discouraging.

There is, for example, the quasi-social worker who has come into existence with some of the community-based programs for old people. Just as the children have their cutesy-pie Head Start, the aged have their equally cute Second Start, Late Start, SCORE, FIND, SERVE, AIDE, Green Thumb, Green Light, etc., ad nauseam. One such worker I met spent the first five minutes of every single interview saying, "I just love my old people. They're so *cute!* I just *love* them. And they love me."

If anyone ever had occasion to call her before 11 A.M., she was not at the program center, because she was "out late with a client" the night before. (This excuse always gave people a fleeting picture of the lady out dancing the rhumba with an octogenarian.) Maybe they drank too much, also, because she always talked compulsively as if she were just getting over a drunk. The major target of her talk was the "real" social worker, who didn't really care about old people: "Oh, I'm not saying anything against her, you understand. But she just doesn't know . . . know . . . uh. . . ."

The "real" social worker's tendency to talk a little too much has over the years solidified into pontification, since her ideas are solidly rooted in a professional degree. When she is asked about recreational activities in the center for old people that she runs, she is rather vague about everything except that they have a whole house that they bought after many tribulations and contributions. She also presents questioners with a dollop of weighty opinion:

"I don't like old people watching television. It's not reality."

She promises to send the center station wagon to pick an old man up in the afternoons and drive him back for a game of chess or some conversation with some of the old people who come to the center. The station wagon never shows up.

When the man's son calls to ask why, she says they really don't provide that service; she was just doing it as a favor. And anyway, there weren't any activities at the center at this time of year.

The old man's physician, a specialist in gerontology, lauds the center and the social worker who runs it. (She has named one of the rooms after him, in recognition of the good work he does with old people.) He offers to write her a note asking her to see what she can do to provide some diversion for his patient.

Again the old man's son goes to the center. And again the social worker is sitting behind the same desk. He gets the same pronouncement about television, the same promise to pick up his father, and the same failure to do so.

In asking around the community, the son was never able to locate one old person who ever found his way to the recreation room of the center, although he met many concerned people who had contributed money at various times to support the center and its programs.

Reading Coleman's statement about England, Scotland, and Wales, that "Too few services are actually planned on the basis of the need which exists," [19] brings to mind the case of Hannah Weiss, who fell victim to one man's drive to serve.

He's called a friendly visitor and he prides himself on all the good he does for the people he visits—some old, some infirm. Hannah always, when they met, had the almost-irresistible urge to remind him that he got paid for visiting—paid at the prevailing fair-wage standard. The urge was precipitated by his officious condescension when he talked about the people he visited. So "friendly" was he that he called the people "my clients," ludicrously adopting the jargon of the social workers who "supervised" him, and successfully communicating that friendliness was certainly not the basis of his service to them.

He bolstered his image of himself as "one who serves" by gossiping about the infirmities of his "clients"—always with an overlay of expressed pity to illustrate how, without him, those poor people would be bereft and abandoned.

When he first came to Hannah's home, he looked about and began to make suggestions for improving the quality of the visit: "You have candy—for when we sit around?" he asked Hannah.

"Candy?" She had not eaten candy since she was a teenager. She was now 82.

"Yes. I can't eat chocolate, but other kinds of candy are good."

"Of course. Candy." She made a note to buy some.

"What time do you eat lunch?" he asked.

"Lunch. Oh, about 12 o'clock. Long before you come. You'll be coming at 1:00, won't you?"

"I'm often out with the blind in the morning. I take them where they want to go. So I have to eat afterward."

"My daughter prepares my lunch before she leaves. She leaves it in the refrigerator for me."

"I have your daughter's number at work. I'll call her."

"What is it you want to talk to her about? Maybe I can help you."

"I just want to tell her. I'll talk to her."

Without another word and without a by-your-leave he went to the phone, obviously well on the way to arranging his friendly visit to suit *his* needs. The ringing phone interrupted Hannah's daughter's work, something the mother would not bring herself to do if she were in imminent danger of expiring.

"Miss Weiss, I just wanted to tell you."

"Is my mother all right?!"

"I just wanted to tell you that I'll bring a sandwich to eat."

"What?"

"I take the blind people in the morning and I'll bring a sandwich."

"Uh, er fine."

"Your mother eats her lunch at 12 o'clock."

"Yes."

"I'll be here a little earlier. I'll bring a sandwich."

"Fine."

"I don't want to impose, but do you mind if I make myself a cup of tea?"

"No, No. That's all right. Anything you want."

"I didn't want to take anything without asking you."

"That's all right. Let me talk to my mother."

"Maybe some candy for when we sit around."

"Put my mother on the phone, please."

Mrs. Weiss came to the phone, anxious and troubled. "Jen, I'm sorry."

"It's all right, Ma. Don't worry about it. He just wanted me to say I'd prepare lunch for him, too. But I'm damned if I will. He's supposed to make things easier for us, not give us more work to do."

"Maybe we should, Jen. Maybe. . . ."

"Mom, remember. He works for us. Don't let him convince you that you're an object of charity. He's there to take you where you want to go, to help you carry a package. And he's paid for it. Don't let him make you feel that you owe him anything before you even get to know each other."

"You know best, Jen. Whatever you say."

"Goodbye, Mom. Have a nice afternoon."

Jen Weiss hung up the phone and cursed into the air. Damn it to hell if I'll do any extra shopping or preparing for a friendly visitor! That's why I arranged for afternoon visits—to avoid meals. I need *less* work—not more!

Thus, in ways subtle and not so subtle, the urge to serve is tempered by the belief that the serving should be done almost exclusively on the server's terms. The person in charge of the recreation center for older people tells you, "Bring your father in at 10 o'clock. If there's no one here, you can bring him back later." And who feeds you when you lose your job because you're walking your father back and forth between home and the center?

"I became an L.P.N. because I wanted to help people," says the middle-aged lady who comes into your home to help bathe and dress your mother. "When I see someone like this—so helpless—I just want to help."

"My mother is quite able to understand, and even to help herself a little. Aren't you mother?"

"Yes. They told us in training that the hearing is often the last sense to go."

"Will you please stop talking about my mother as if she weren't here!"

"Well, there are plenty of people who appreciate what I do for them. I really give everything to my old people."

"Go away! Go to the people who appreciate you!"

And you are left to bathe and dress your mother by yourself— another desperate attempt to save her sense of dignity.

The physician who writes the prescription but won't listen to the questions. The nurse who won't use the social and psychological information on her own nursing history to change her care plan. The social worker who will give you a list of facilities but never visit one to assess the quality of service provided. Although they may not be typical or in the majority in the profession (we do not have that data), they lend their coloration sufficiently to make many people reluctant to seek service, and even hostile when they are compelled to accept it.

This is a dreary picture of people in the service professions. It needs balancing, I know. Perhaps the findings of one British researcher give indications of what we might find here, too [20]:

> Of particular interest in British research in this field in recent years are controlled studies of the effects of particular types of social provisions for the elderly. Most notable has been Goldberg's . . . praiseworthy

study to assess the effectiveness of social work with the elderly. The methods employed by social workers, their objectives and the effectiveness of their efforts, were investigated among a group of 300 old people aged 70 and over who were all applicants to a London borough welfare department. Their social and medical condition and needs were assessed by a social worker and a physician beforehand. Half the group were randomly selected to receive help from trained case workers (who gave them more time and attention and made a greater effort to enrich their lives by introducing them to clubs, voluntary agencies, and family connections), while the other half remained with experienced local authority welfare officers without professional training. The social and medical conditions of the surviving clients were reassessed after nearly a year. Both sets of social workers had achieved much in alleviating practical needs, but the trained workers had brought about more change in their clients' activities, feelings, and attitudes. More of them had attended clubs, had had a holiday, felt satisfied with life, and had fewer worries.

The Nurse as Patient Advocate

Nurses are in a strategic position to intercede on behalf of patients who need advocacy in a situation where other professionals seem insensitive to their needs. In whatever setting she functions, the nurse can bring her accurate information about old people, her awareness of the margin for error in the perceptions of many other professionals, and her skills in communication to protect the patient from the corrosive effects of prejudice and discrimination. In addition, she can institute and maintain a program of informal education that will help to reduce the error and increase awareness and sensitivity.

In the hospital setting, the registered nurse is usually in a position of supervision and/or administration, so that, by definition, her role must include taking the leadership in setting and maintaining standards of professional behavior. Here, she is in a position to:

1. model appropriate behavior vis-à-vis old people

They key to model behavior might be to help the old person maintain a sense of control over his own life. Unless he is completely unaware of his surroundings, his whole conception of self is affected when all decisions concerning his own body are made by others. It is questionable that this is always a necessary qualification for therapeutic outcomes.

Early in his professional education, the nurse is taught as a basic precept that patients are to be helped to independent functioning as quickly as is consistent with good therapeutic procedures. This goal of patient independence has a great many implications for effective interaction with old people. When young people feel that they have no power to change the course of events in their lives, when they feel that they are merely the targets of a capricious fate, they are unable to initiate any action to improve their lives. They feel that, no matter what they do, they will be unsuccessful in changing anything.

The old person in the hospital may be similarly affected when the professionals who surround her efficiently organize her time and control her body functions. The knowledgeable and sensitive nurse is able to draw the patient into the deliberations and the decision making about how her life in the hospital is to be managed. Knowing as he does the importance of independent functioning—even for old people—and resistant as he is to the stereotype of the aged as incompetent and childish, he takes the time to come to a mutual agreement with the patient on a satisfactory division of control, making it clear that, as the patient's condition improves, she will assume more control over her own life.

What the old person certainly does *not* need is additional evidence from the world around her that she is not considered worthwhile as a human being. Complete takeover of her management when she is able to maintain at least a part of it is calculated to make her feel useless. The good nurse knows that a person who feels useless and unworthy will not be able to learn much, because she believes that her unworthy self is not deserving of the effort learning takes. She also feels quite sure that any effort to learn is wasted because the only possible outcome is failure.

For many patients, a failure to learn is tantamount to extended and exacerbated illness and even death. Certainly, with old people, among whom the incidence of chronic illness is higher than for other age groups, acquiring new information and skills for management of illness is very important.

The nurse can help make the stay in the hospital for the old person an excitingly revelatory experience, during which she begins to see herself as capable and worthy of self-respect. For the other workers who come into contact with the patient and have occasion to observe the way the nurse functions, the experience can be just as illuminating, and have the effect of changing for the better a pattern of interaction with old people in the hospital.

2. see that standards of behavior for the staff are defined and put in writing

We long ago learned in intergroup relations that there is no substitute for a written statement of policy against which behavior in an institution may be checked and evaluated. Such a written statement helps employees to maintain fair practices. It also is often useful for shifting responsibility for resisting discrimination to the institution, thereby taking the onus off an individual in a difficult situation. For example, if a patient 30 years old complains to an attendant that he does not want an octogenarian brought in to share his room, the attendant need not argue about the matter. She need only say that the hospital policy is clear: there is to be no segregation on the basis of age. (Is it too soon in our development as a culture to suggest that this should apply to children, also?)

If the standards are clearly delineated and made known to all employees, no one can take it on himself to decide *how much* discrimination should be practiced. Thus, although it is difficult to make operable merely by edict a rule that old people are not to be treated as if they were children, a clear statement that old men are not to be addressed as "Pops" can easily be monitored and enforced.

Similarly, written standards for the treatment of old people may include:

a. The word "crock" is not to be used in the hospital to refer to a patient (just as proscriptions against the use of racial epithets are, I think, justifiable).

b. Every adult patient is to be addressed by title unless he states a preference for the use of his given name, in which case he is to be encouraged to use the given name of the employee. If the employee prefers to be called by title, then he must use the patient's title. (This may, on the surface, seem trivial to some people, or even a misconstruction of motive, but the issue has gone to the courts in the case of white people who used given names when addressing black people to make clear the differences in status between them. Equal status communication cannot be maintained with differential forms of address.)

c. Patients over 65 are to have their questions answered in the same way that we answer the questions of younger adults. (It is not to be assumed that information about older patients should go only to younger members of their families.)

d. Restraints are not to be used on anyone until all possible alternatives have been explored with the patient, his family, and the members of the health team. (Tying a patient to his bed is too often rationalized as being for the patient's good—for his safety, for his health, for his comfort. When a patient is confused or feeble, it sometimes seems as if the rationalization is applied too quickly and too broadly, almost as if the patient's limited ability to resist makes this "remedy" easier to use. When I consider the essential violation that restraints represent, and when I remember the weeping and groaning and pulling and writhing of patients who were tied down, I would explore every other possibility before I would use them. No—I would go further with this: I would not use them under any circumstances. I have heard too often the excuse that, "He doesn't really mind; he doesn't know what's happening," even while the patient continues to struggle and his agitation increases.)

The ultimate alternative is to have a constant watch kept on the patient who keeps wandering off the bed or pulling the IV from his arm. One reason why this is not done is that *it costs too much money!* Weighing in the balance the look of pain on the faces and the outlay of money, I find it easy to make a choice.

But there are other ways to provide constant vigilance when it is needed. The reason we think there is not is because we always have close at hand the simple expedient of forcible restraint. As in the search for solutions to international problems, as long as war is a viable alternative, we search so far, but no further. If war were absolutely out of the question, we would continue to search until we found newer and more creative solutions.

Putting the patient who needs watching in a room with many other people so that someone can alert the staff when necessary is one way. Putting the patient in the corridor near the nurse's station is another way. We have patients in the hallways when hospitals are crowded— why not one patient in the hallway to save him some suffering? We can even encourage a family and neighbors to set up a round-the-clock vigil until the patient no longer needs watching.

I think the extra effort is worthwhile; tying a human being down is no trivial matter.

3. develop and operate a pattern of supervision to maintain a high quality of functioning

A *sine qua non* of effective supervision of service workers is input from the recipients of the service. Any plan for supervision must have built into it systematic feedback from patients and family members as well as from the workers themselves. The feedback system must be open, and the information must be freely discussed with all parties involved so that there does not develop a situation of spying and secretive tale-bearing that will only result in a lower quality of work.

Patients and personnel must be clear about the objectives of the total supervisory system, and efforts should be made to help each person recognize the benefits to him from participating in the process.

It occurs to me that the health team as described by me earlier [21] would be an ideal format for monitoring the behavior of hospital personnel toward old people. The open setting, with optimum involvement of all hospital personnel who have contact with the patient, the freedom to raise questions and provide information, can result in a gradual and systematic discarding of archaic stereotypes and inappropriate behaviors.

As an adjunct to the regular team functioning, instruments similar to the "Self-Check on Beliefs About Aging" in Chapter 3, the "Checklist of Ambivalent Behaviors" in Chapter 2, and the "Forty-Five Questions To Ask on the Job" in Chapter 6 can be used by individuals to keep track of the quality of their own interaction.

4. institute a formal program of in-service education

The nursing profession, perhaps more than any other of the health professions, is committed to regular in-service education. Generally, however, the programs are attended only by nurses, and the advantages of on-site study by all personnel involved with a group of patients are lost. The result often is some consensus among nurses on behavior and standards of operation, and dissemination of up-to-date information among *them*. But in the day-to-day job functions, much energy is dissipated and much frustration generated in the efforts to make other personnel work as if they had shared in developing the standards and accepted them, and as if they, too, were privy to the latest data.

5. extend communication about standards of behavior toward old people and information about age and aging to those professionals who are generally outside her supervision network

It is unfortunate that physicians continue to remain aloof from whatever struggles nurses engage in against archaic modes of thinking and behavior. Similarly, technicians and other personnel who come into regular contact with patients are in a position to nullify the progress nurses make in the quality of their relationships with old people. Everyone should be included in the communication network through which standards of operation and new data are disseminated.

Obviously, nursing supervisors and administrators may not always be able to compel personnel outside their jurisdiction to attend education programs or health-team meetings. But they can encourage such personnel to participate. There are other methods that might be tried to extend the communication network. The one used most often, of course, is regularly sending out written announcements and informational flyers. Unfortunately, if too many of these are received, they are often discarded without being read. In addition, the danger of written notices is that— unless they are thoroughly discussed—they may be misunderstood and subjectively interpreted.

A way of dealing with these dangers is to encourage a pattern of open observation of all patient-personnel interaction. That is, when someone in the supervision network—an R.N., or an aide, or an attendant —hears an X-ray technician shouting his directions to an old person, she may repeat a direction in a normal tone of voice and so illustrate that shouting is not necessary. Or she may, calmly and pleasantly, offer the information that Mr. Smith's hearing is unimpaired. To help the technician save face, she may suggest that he is probably confusing Mr. Smith with another patient. If this sort of observation and comment is done consistently, the pattern of interaction with old people will inevitably change as the consciousness of all personnel is raised.

In the physician's office, the nurse can set the tone of optimal interaction with the old person. She can take time before and after his examination by the doctor to

1. develop an ambience of relaxed use of time

Relaxed use of time is quite different from just keeping someone waiting for a long time. After waiting for an hour or two, it is disconcerting, to say the least, to have the doctor spend fifteen minutes with you, only half listening to your answers to his cursory questions while he examines you. If long waits are really unavoidable—and I am not at all sure that they are—the time spent waiting can be used to achieve viable therapeutic objectives. (See items 2, 3, 4, and 5.)

The process, however, is quite different from the traditional one of seating the patient beside a desk and filling out a form as he responds to prepared questions. There is nothing relaxed about this process, focused as it is on "processing" patients in turn. In addition, the tension created in this kind of controlled situation often makes people respond in ways that are not quite accurate. Whether the reason is inability to recall accurately, or the felt pressure to complete the questionnaire, or the need to make a certain kind of impression on the questioner, the total information gathered is not as useful as the information given in a less formal, more relaxed atmosphere.

The semisocial interchange when the nurse sits in the waiting room chatting with three or four patients may produce significant information of the kind that people are more likely to reveal to acquaintances and friends than they are to doctors and nurses. It also offers opportunity for patients to share some general expectations and anxieties and so alleviate the special tension that arises out of the belief that one is all alone in his misery.

If the nurse's duties in the office involve her more technical professional skills, she can educate the receptionist to take over this function, arming her with the kinds of questions and comments that are calculated to encourage certain types of communication. The ringing phone and the bill typing can be reserved for those times when the doctor has no visiting hours.

2. find out something about his expectations and anxieties

An opening gambit may establish the informality and make it clear that there are no taboo feelings or thoughts. The nurse may reveal something about her own anxiety in a similar situation and so encourage the patient's expression of feeling. One nurse tested this process by coming out from behind the partition that separated her office from the waiting room and offering lemonade to the two old people sitting there so patiently. After sitting down with them for a moment or two, she observed, "Do you know, when I've been waiting for a long time to see a doctor, I begin to wonder about all the other people on his mind, and all their ailments. I can't help feeling that I'd better not take up too much of his time with my little aches and pains. Then after I leave, I'm sorry that I didn't mention this or that, and it bothers me until my next visit."

One of the patients responded, "He always seems to be so busy. It makes me nervous, trying to get out what I want to say."

The other patient smiled sympathetically, "I used to stutter when I was younger. Now the only time I do is when I'm talking to the doctor. I try to talk fast."

The nurse was able to provide information that might alleviate the apparent tension the patients felt by telling them, "The doctor plans for a full forty minutes for you on routine visits. That's more than enough time to talk to him about what's on your mind. And if anything special comes up, he's told me to just help the people who are waiting to be comfortable. So I know he hopes you'll just relax and talk to him as we're talking now."

3. encourage him to put into words whatever questions he has

Sometimes, if the old person has had opportunity to verbalize some questions on his mind, he can get answers in the informal situation that are satisfactory and leave him free to communicate with the physician about more immediately relevant medical matters. One such patient, encouraged by the trained receptionist, asked, "What is leukocyst?" "Leukocyst. I don't know such a word. Maybe you mean leucocyte?" "What is it?" "A white blood cell," she answered. "Oh," said the patient, obviously enlightened and relieved. "When I went to the lab for tests, they kept talking about it, and I couldn't imagine what it was. I thought I had a rare disease."

Although I have no hard data on this, I would venture to say that receptionists behind glass, or even behind desks, are not often asked questions like this. And, on the rare occasions when they are, the patient is rebuffed by an admonition to save such questions for the doctor. If the patient feels constrained to respond only minimally to the doctor, then he is inevitably left with many unanswered questions that contribute unnecessarily to his discomfort.

4. make some obvious efforts to see her as a whole person

The work she did before retiring can still be drawn on for interest and self-concept maintenance. It is good to continue to get recognition for activity that once defined your whole life. The request for an opinion about the current political campaign or a local labor dispute makes it clear that the old person is still considered to be tuned in to what is happening around him and is as concerned as any younger person might be. (There is evidence that a significant number of old people are even *more* concerned about political events than are many younger people!)

A new movie or play, a best-selling book—how many younger people discuss these things with old people with whom they come into contact? It is no wonder that young people so often think that association with the old is dull; they assume that old people are not interested in the things that young people think about.

5. interact productively with the friend, paid companion, or family member who accompanies the patient

The person who accompanies an old man or woman to the doctor's office has valuable information that may help the nurse and the doctor treat the patient more successfully. Unfortunately, however, there is often a tendency to talk to this person *about* the old person as if the latter were not present. The sensitive nurse can change the pattern of interaction by making it a three-way affair and, in the process, perhaps teach another adult to change a destructive form of behavior.

Sometimes an altogether different attitude seems to manifest itself toward an adult son or daughter of an old person. Doctors and nurses could do much to alleviate the anxieties and frustrations of adults who must suddenly assume the care of aged parents who can no longer care for themselves. However, they often seem unaware of the need for such help and may even thoughtlessly exacerbate the difficulties with some of the things they say and do—or do *not* say and do.

For example, there is a fear that is generated by the TV-perpetuated myth of the good old family doctor who knew you as a child and calls your mother by her given name (as she does his), and stops to have a cup of tea after a home visit to treat a mild cold.

The physician who treats your old mother these days is a very busy man. He can see her—after long waiting—when she is relatively well, or suffering from a persistent, chronic condition for which he needs to renew the medicine. The pervasive dread of the patient's family is that she will suddenly become acutely ill and need a physician immediately. There is no physician for this situation; there are only fire-department medics, hospital emergency rooms, or police wagons. Since one has no way of knowing if the symptoms are only alarming and not really serious, one may get involved with the whole emergency apparatus, including crowds in front of the house, and scare the old woman and the rest of the family half to death, when all that was needed was a simple remedy and some reassurance. No geriatrist ever seems to raise the matter with the family, and, somehow, one feels that talking about it would be an imposition on his time and his professional sophistication. He has more important things to do than respond to the fears of his patient's family—doesn't he?

An adult daughter cannot help remembering that once her father became ill when he lived alone, and nobody knew about it for hours. So now that he lives with her, she finds herself getting up several times during the night to see that he is all right, like a new mother with her child. Each nocturnal trip he makes to the bathroom, she listens to his footsteps, and turns back to sleep only when he is safe in bed again. When the night turns cold, she gets up to see if he has remembered where the extra blanket is, or, if the weather is warm, that he remembers how to open the sliding window; she doesn't want him catching cold. Aren't old people more susceptible to colds than younger people? (How is it that she forgets so completely that her father hasn't had a cold in twenty years, and she's had *three* since he's come to live with her?)

Most parents who respond to their infants this way learn to relax and be less fearful as time goes on. The pediatrician knows this and keeps telling the new parents that it will happen to them, too. Most fears prove to be groundless, and children are manifestly hardy survivors. But the geriatrist doesn't seem to recognize that it is difficult to develop this perspective about an old person. He so often does have aches and pains that make him as fearful as they make his family.

Has a nurse or physician ever asked a son or daughter how he feels about having a parent live with him? Just a recognition by professionals that there *are* feelings may help that person do better by the parent, and so influence the ultimate therapeutic objective.

6. institute a process of informal education about old age and aging

The nurse can initiate a process of education to reduce stereotypic thinking and discriminatory behavior against old people. But the program in the physician's office will probably need to be an informal one, although there is no reason why it cannot be as carefully planned and systematically executed as any formal in-service program.

The nurse can suggest to all the other personnel—including the physician—that they all watch for evidences of errors in thinking about old people and post a description of each error (without identifying the person who erred) on a bulletin board. If the target is one error a week, the nurse can encourage informal discussion of that error—at lunch, during coffee breaks, and during other moments of casual conversation—and bring to each discussion some information or observation calculated to increase knowledge about old age and aging and awareness of the needs of old people.

Selected readings can be brought into the office and left in strategic spots where personnel may pick them up. Lectures, TV shows, and other presentations of data about aging can be brought to everybody's attention, and discussions about them can be initiated on the following day. The results of the informal gathering of data from old people (see item 1) can be shared with technicians and receptionists, who do not ordinarily have access to patient histories, so that the pitfalls of stereotyping can be pinpointed in specific cases.

In the community-based health care agency, the nurse may define a new role for himself, adding to the traditional professional functions activities and initiatives that may ultimately make nurses the leaders in health-care delivery. Here, the nurse may:

1. learn to read the living text that is the community

More and more, health-care delivery is moving out of the traditional offices and institutions and into the community. No generalizations gleaned from lectures and textbooks can substitute for the living unfolding of events, the everyday evidences of attitudes, and the immediate effect of behaviors that every community uniquely presents.

In some communities, there are many old people who are rearing their grandchildren while parents work or are just absent. These old people need the kind of day-to-day help that agencies for "senior citizens" never seem to provide. They need up-to-date information on child care, lessons on nutrition for growing children as well as for themselves, and help in providing for immunization. They are concerned about lead-paint poisoning and other dangers to children, and they should have opportunity to meet with young parents, not only with old people.

In other communities, three generations of families live in houses near each other. Often, the old people move in with one of the sons and daughters. Here the medical/psychological/social needs that might be identified by a community nurse would include meetings of all generations to discuss problems of health that arise when living with someone who suffers from a chronic illness, or who has certain debilities that necessitate physical changes in the house, or who has introduced a dimension of interaction that is causing trouble with children or with a spouse.

In still other communities, old people live alone, and they often need a system of regular checks to see if they require assistance of one kind or another.

The point is that the nurse in the health-care agency does not know what the community's needs are if she does not talk to the people, visit them, or work with them in their community efforts. And if the nurse does not know the needs, the chances are that the other health personnel will not be learning those needs. It is the nurse whose professional education provides some impetus for acquiring knowledge of the patient as a whole person.

Often the community health center employs people from the community to work in various staff capacities. In this case, the nurse has an opportunity to establish the kind of atmosphere in which "nonprofessionals" are recognized as having valuable information and insights to contribute to the process of planning for community needs. They know, better than any outsider, how the old people in the community live.

2. protect individual old people from community neglect and mistreatment

When the outside professional is trusted by the community, pipelines are run to him carrying all kinds of information and cries for help. The nurse who is recognized by everyone when she walks down a street, the nurse who is greeted by the children and stopped by the housewife to answer a question about Johnny's bruise, will also learn about the old man who is being harassed by the children on their way home from school, and about the old woman who had a fight with her daughter and is now abandoned to shift for herself. When that old man and that old woman come to the agency for medical treatment, the nurse has additional information for diagnosing the etiology of the increased hand tremors or the sharp drop in red cell count. She can help in the treatment of the whole person rather than of isolated symptoms.

Nurses are often the ones who are asked for advice by family members and by old people about what to do when problems of living proliferate. The agitation sometimes seems far greater than the problems seem to warrant, given the available resources and the possible alternative solutions, and the nurse who knows her community can defuse the agitation with a knowledgeable, skillful, problem-solving approach.

Above all, she learns to avoid telling people just what they ought to do—a common error made by professionals who have learned all their answers in academic or academically cushioned settings, like large teaching hospitals. In the community, she learns that—professional or not— her knowledge and her skill will not be used unless she is trusted, unless she makes it clear that she respects the knowledge and insights of the community, and unless she is ready to accept that the community knows better than any outsider what it needs. Only then can she be of real help—especially to those whom the community victimizes by mistreatment and neglect.

3. institute a program of education for the younger people in the community to improve their attitudes and behavior toward old people

The nurse who makes himself available in a community to answer questions pertaining to health may soon find himself in the midst of planning for regular sessions dealing with health areas of concern to the community. Every such session can include some material on attitude toward and treatment of old people.

In a seminar on sex, the myths perpetuated about the asexuality of the old may be dissipated. The special dangers to old people of broken sidewalks and garbage underfoot might be part of discussions about the city's neglect of cleanliness and safety. In campaigning for the immunization of children, some of the special immunization needs of the aged might also be broached.

If the old people in a community are forever considered as just another part of the concerned population in a quest for health, and always included in the discussions of needs, the total population begins to accept the idea that "the aged" do not constitute an alien, extra "cohort," with needs that cut in on the needs of the rest of the community.

Notes

1. David Guttman, Francis L. Eyster, and Garland Lewis, *The Gerontologist*, Vol. 15, No. 5, Part 1, October, 1975, pp. 387–392.

2. Ibid., quoting M. I. Brown, "Nursing of the Aging and the Aged," Section with aspects special to the allied health professions, Part XVII, Nursing, *Working With Older People*, Vol. 12, PHS Publication No. 1459, July, 1971.

3. Ibid., quoting John Bullock and John W. Bauman Jr., "Gerontology in Medical Education: An Elective Program in Research and Training," *The Gerontologist*, Vol. 14, No. 14, August, 1974, pp. 319–323.

4. Donald Kent, "Aging: Fact and Fantasy," *The Gerontologist*, Vol. 5, No. 2, June, 1965, pp. 51–56, 111.

5. Ibid.

6. Robert C. Atchley, *The Social Forces in Later Life,* Wadsworth Publishing Co., Inc., Belmont, Calif., 1972, p. 127.

7. Ibid., pp. 62–63.

8. John E. Anderson, "Environment and Meaningful Activity," in Richard H. Williams, Clark Tibbits, and Wilma Donahue, *Processes of Aging,* Vol. I, Atherton Press, New York, 1963, pp. 223–245.

9. Ibid.

10. Rose, op. cit.

11. Charlotte Epstein, *Nursing the Dying Patient,* Reston Publishing Company, Reston, Va., 1975, p. 91.

12. Bartram B. Moss, with Kent Fraser, *Caring for the Aged,* Doubleday & Company, Inc., New York, 1966, p. 131.

13. Peter Coleman, "Social Gerontology in England, Scotland, and Wales; A Review of Recent and Current Research," *The Gerontologist,* Vol. 15, No. 3, June, 1975, pp. 219–229.

14. Atchley, op. cit., p. 7.

15. Ibid., pp. 26–27.

16. Natalie Harris Cabot, *You Can't Count on Dying,* Houghton Mifflin Company, Boston, 1961, p. 254.

17. Moss, op. cit., p. 136.

18. Division of Research and Analysis, Office of Research, Demonstrations and Manpower Resources, Administration on Aging, Office of Human Development; Department of Health, Education, and Welfare, *Research and Development Strategy,* Fiscal Year 1975.

19. Coleman, op. cit.

20. Ibid.

21. Charlotte Epstein, *Effective Interaction in Contemporary Nursing,* Prentice-Hall, Inc., Englewood Cliffs, N.J., 1974, pp. 124–147.

6

*exercises in awareness
and skill development*

*identifying job factors
in nursing the aged*

Forty-Five Questions to Ask on the Job

1. At what age does the staff believe a person is old?
2. What does the staff believe all old people have in common?
3. Is there a procedure or part of a procedure to which all old people in the hospital are subjected?
4. Are old people generally assigned rooms with other old people?
5. What are behaviors appropriate to old age that the staff agrees on?
6. Does the staff generally agree that it is qualified to give advice on the life-styles of old people?
7. Is there a mandatory retirement age?
8. Are any other factors besides age to be considered in forced retirement?
9. Are there volunteers in the institution who are considered old?
10. What are the factors considered in identifying them as old?
11. Does the staff offer advice to old people and their families in areas they feel is none of their business when dealing with younger people?
12. Does the staff generally believe that old people need to be told what to do and how to live more often than younger people do?
13. Do younger people get explanations about medical procedure more readily and more fully than old people do?
14. Are there some things done for young people that the staff thinks are not necessary for old people, such as stopping in to chat about current community events?
15. Does the staff generally decide on meals for old people rather than take the trouble to question them as to their prefrences if they have some difficulty in filling out menus by themselves?
16. Does the staff take steps to find out how the old people who are patients feel about being in the hospital?
17. Does the staff take steps to know how the old people feel about being ill?
18. Does the staff ever discuss old age, death, and dying with patients who are old?
19. Does the staff call all old people by their first names without ascertaining their preference?
20. Does the staff ask old people to call *them* by their first names?
21. Do staff members ever talk to other staff members on behalf of the patient who is old?
22. Do staff members at all ranks feel free to talk to staff members of higher ranks about the needs of patients who are old?
23. Are old people pressured—subtly and not-so-subtly—to submit to procedures before they really understand them?

24. Are families of old people—rather than the patients themselves—approached more often for consent to procedures than are families of younger people?

25. Is more time spent by the staff with younger patients than with older patients?

26. Does the term "senile" appear on patients' histories and charts?

27. Does the staff generally feel that old patients are not able to learn much about new ways to eat and exercise and live?

28. Does the staff demonstrate affection and just human interaction by touching old people?

29. Are old people permitted to have some personal belongings around them in the hospital?

30. Is bathing for old people considered a private function by the staff?

31. Is eating for old people considered a social function by the staff?

32. Does the staff treat rich old people differently from the way they treat poor old people?

33. Does the staff treat white old people differently from the way they treat Black old people?

34. Does the staff treat old English-speaking people differently from the way they treat old people who speak other languages?

35. Is there explicit machinery that old people know about and that they may use to change what they consider discriminatory treatment by staff?

36. Are there regular in-service courses for all the staff on interacting with the aged?

37. Has the staff ever sat and talked about the *positive* factors of being old?

38. Is a psychiatrist consulted for aged patients for the same reasons that he is consulted for younger patients?

39. Are physical symptoms of old people explored as carefully as are similar symptoms of young people?

40. Are staff members more polite to old patients than they are to younger patients?

41. Are staff members vociferously admiring of old patients but not of younger patients?

42. Do staff members believe that they are entirely different from the old people who are patients?

43. Do staff members believe that patients who are old are generally less cooperative than younger patients?

44. Does the staff think that patients who are old are more demanding of their time and energies than younger patients are?

45. Do staff members believe that patients who are old need befriending more often than younger patients do?

As I suggested earlier, questions about attitudes and behaviors of health personnel may be raised in team meetings, where any team member should be able to voice a particular concern.

As part of an in-service education program, clusters of questions may be used as a basis for planning and systematic study. An aspect of such study could be data gathering on attitudes and practices, as well as a search for additional information from scientific resources.

In a less formal but nonetheless systematic way, a small group of staff members might be polled to see if they have one or two common areas of interest or concern. For example, they may all agree that they have observed a behavior vis-à-vis patients who are old that they object to as demeaning and destructive. They may then get together to attempt to find effective ways to eliminate this behavior.

They might begin with brainstorming, a process designed to start the creative juices flowing. The people sit around a table, each with a stack of about twenty small cards or pieces of paper. A time limit of about five minutes is set, and at the word "Go," the group members write —one idea to a card—every possible way that occurs to them to solve the problem. They are *not* to think through each method carefully. Rather, they are to write uncritically, and as quickly as possible, with the objective of accumulating as many ideas as they can, no matter how impractical or bizarre. As they finish each card, they are to toss it in the center of the table, so that no one need be identified with the idea if he prefers not to be.

When the time allotted is up, the cards are shuffled, and the group examines each idea, discussing it, bringing additional information and insights to bear on it, discarding parts of it, adding new dimensions, or discarding it completely. Sometimes, several ideas are combined to provide a single workable one.

Finally, the group makes a decision to try one or more of the ideas, plans exactly how to do it, and sets a time for meeting again to assess progress and amend the plan.

Sometimes a staff—or part of a staff—can select one question to work on for a designated period of time. During that time, people keep asking the questions of each other and inviting responses based on their most recent experience. This can be done quickly, just in passing, over coffee, almost as quickly as it takes to respond to "Good morning. How are you?" It serves to raise consciousness about a particular attitude and focus on the resultant behaviors. It is almost impossible to maintain an undesirable behavior in so much public light. And just about when people feel they have had enough of it, it is time to go on to another question.

Humanistic Psychology and Health Care Delivery

If professionals often think in stereotypic terms about old people and react to them in ambivalent and discriminatory ways, we must look not only to our total culture, which teaches and reinforces such thinking and behavior; the process of professional education and the structure of professional institutions are also responsible for perpetuating prejudice and discrimination.

We might start with the premise that authoritarianism is antagonistic to humanism. Authoritarianism is characterized by rigidity, exclusiveness, dichotomous thinking, and prejudice. A commitment to the status quo and a resistance to change, which are essential elements of rigidity, when applied to the relationship of the old to the younger, results in accepting as axiomatic that retirement from work is necessary for all, that a benevolent paternalism is the most desirable basis for interacting with the old, and that old people prefer to live with "their own kind."

Exclusiveness fosters the practice of keeping the old from participation in the decision making that affects their lives. It surrounds medical knowledge and medical practice with an aura of mystery, and implies strongly that there is no point in explaining because only the inner circle can understand and appreciate.

Those who view the world in dichotomous terms tend to see most groups as "them" and one's own group as "us." The implication is generally that "they" are inferior to "us," less able to benefit from the advantages in life. Most things, according to the dichotomous thinker, are either good or bad, right or wrong, for or against. He finds it difficult to see, for example, that any good can be derived from the process of dying or that there are alternatives in old age to resignation and withdrawal.

Prejudice leads one into the error of thinking that all old people are alike, and one has only to listen to the succession of younger adults who raise their voices several decibels whenever they speak to an old person— whether they know him or not, whether they have any evidence that he is hard of hearing or not, whether they know that they need extra sound to get his attention or not—to realize that they are not taking the trouble to check and see if *this* old person really conforms to the picture they have in their minds of *all* old people.

The question is: What does all of this have to do with the practitioners in the health sciences? Physicians, nurses, physical therapists, and other students in the field are systematically trained in authoritarianism. They make, generally, little or no contribution to the development of programs in which they are students. The pattern of teaching is generally one of sitting and taking the notes of lectures by authorities in the field. As students, they are generally so frightened and intimidated by their teachers, other staff, and the constant threat of failure that—from what we know about the psychology of learning—it is an amazing testimony to their resiliency that they learn as much as they do.

After they finish their formal schooling, their internships and residencies continue to be characterized by relationships that are authoritarian. There is a rigid hierarchy of roles in most clinical situations and an etiquette between "ranks" that precludes optimum communication. Between supervisors and the people they supervise the dominance/submissive relationship perpetuates the educational pattern. In subtle and not-so-subtle ways, the authoritarian respect for power and strength is manifested in the clinical setting. Ultimately, patients also are forced into this pattern of interaction with the practitioner. Things are done *to* them, too often without consultation or explanation. The rationalization invariably is that these things are done *for* them: doctors and nurses know what must be done for patients; patients don't know about these things and do better when they follow the directions of the medical practitioners. The authoritarian individual always knows what is best for others, or is ready to submit without question to those who purport to know what is best for *him*.

The humanist rejects the belief that the individual should not maintain control over the decisions that affect his own life—his own body. He believes that people are entitled to the opportunity to face reality and deal with it productively. The idea that the medical professional has the right to keep from a person the extent or nature of his illness, the method of treating it, or the information that he does not have long to live is rejected by the humanist.

The essential democratic orientation of the humanist compels him to reject the making of unilateral decisions for people whose lives are affected by those decisions. This does not mean that each patient is approached with brutal frankness, and precipitously and directly told everything there is to be known. There are other modes of communication, and the humanist, committed as he is to optimum communication, takes the time and the trouble to discover what the patient is saying to him in subtle, and sometimes symbolic, ways. And he learns to respond to the needs he discovers.

Medical education does not assist students to resist the effects of living in a society that labels and stereotypes whole groups of people. Nor does it engage in systematic efforts to overcome the stance of indifference to other groups of people. There are still women students and physicians who are subtly harassed by their colleagues and teachers, if, that is, they are admitted to programs of study. And in professions that have been traditionally almost exclusively for women, the men coming into it are often victimized, even if it is only with raised eyebrows and silent reservations about their masculinity.

Prejudice and discrimination against Black students and practitioners pretty much follows the pattern of interaction in the larger society. And discrimination against Black patients is often so outrageously apparent that Black people must carry, in addition to the burden of being hospitalized, the burden of fear that their race will too often determine the quality and the nature of the treatment they get.

As for old people, what other profession has a special derogatory term for the old? The "crock" is known in medicine for his chronic low-level suffering, which he makes known to those who care for him. But he is a "crock," and so viewed with exasperation and treated with reluctance. Nor is there very much in the various courses of professional study that attempts to deal systematically with the attitudes of young people.

Even the definition and treatment of senility (presumably a medical term) becomes a function of stereotyping. It is only recently that some students of the aged are beginning to observe that what have been diagnosed as symptoms of senility may just be signs of maladjustment. The senility label easily becomes justification for minimal medical treatment and social interaction; for all practical purposes the "senile" individual is discarded.

The "maladjustment" label is something of an improvement, because it implies that the symptoms are found in all age groups and so are treatable. However, it is not much of an improvement, since it does what we, as a society, so often do to the victims of our mistreatment: it implies that the fault lies *with* the victim, that *he* is the one who is not responding appropriately. We stereotype the individuals of a whole group, we force them out of roles on which their self-esteem depends, we exclude them not only from participation in life in general but from participation in the very decisions that affect them personally—and then, when they become profoundly depressed and withdrawn, forgetful and vague, weak and overly concerned with body symptoms, we label them senile or, at best, maladjusted.

Medicine as a profession succumbs to the fear of death and dying that characterizes the attitude of most people in our society. In addition, the nature of the healing professions encourages a tendency to view the death of a patient as a professional failure. The societal and the professional attitudes reinforce and compound each other and the effect is the widespread practice of avoiding the dying patient, and trying to keep the fact of his dying from him. Nothing so characterizes antihumanism!

When a person is close to death, he is often left more alone than he has ever been. When he most needs the reassurance of touching another human being, sharing his fears, communicating his sadness, he is treated with strict medical "correctness" and then abandoned to live out his remaining time alone.

Families are drawn into a similar pattern of interaction because they are products of the same social conditioning as the medical people. They get no help from the "experts" in changing their behavior; they just follow their lead, as they do in most things medical.

Physical therapists also often take on the traditional medical/professional stance while they forget an essential and unique aspect of their role. In their relationship with patients, their teaching function is most important in helping the patient toward improved living capability. In spite of our traditional perception of teaching, there is nothing compatible between effective teaching and authoritarianism. If we accept the humanistic idea that learning is becoming—becoming more human—then there can be no good authoritarian teachers. The authoritarian teacher is characterized by his belief that he is the one who knows the answers and that it is his function to give those answers to the students. There is no question of permitting the student to search out his own answers, adapting his style of learning to his own personality. The authoritarian teacher leaves no room for student spontaneity, for student participation in making decisions about his educational program, for student creativity. The teacher sees "efficiency" as an important good that cannot tolerate the "inefficiency" of democratic participation. The authoritarian teacher demands submissiveness from her students, and is herself submissive to the authoritarian demands of her "superiors." Her vision of humanity is narrowed to accommodate her own perception of what people who come to her are like. Since the authoritarian perception is usually distorted by a rigid, dichotomous view of the world, people are generally viewed as stereotypes, and they are forced into categories that violate their individuality.

Physical therapists know very well that the success of their therapy relies heavily on the cooperation of the patient. If the patient sees the attempts at therapy as a violation of their humanness, they will reject the therapy and reduce the chances of improving their health. Yet very few programs in physical therapy emphasize the teaching/learning aspect of therapy and the essential humanism of the teaching function. This gap, taken together with the general tendencies in our society to view old people as unable to learn ("You can't teach an old dog new tricks.") results too often in the decision to abandon attempts at therapy for the old as useless effort.

Even if physical therapists are not so quick to say that it is no use to try to get old people to exercise in certain ways, to keep trying to improve their functioning, to hold a cane this way instead of that way, they say almost nothing to physicians who are reluctant to prescribe physical therapy for the aged. The authoritarian view that it is not the physical therapist's "place" to protest the physician's decision is usually the deciding factor in the decision to say nothing.

Nurses as a group most consistently feel the effects of authoritarian hospital structure and authoritarian physicians. A recent novel [1] tells the story of a society suddenly become telepathic, in which nurses go mad when they discover that the doctors for whom they worked so diligently never gave them a thought, but merely took their service for granted.

This may be overstating the case, but the nursing profession has yet to overthrow completely the traditional shackles of authoritarianism. Many nurses respond to the taking of orders, the absence of democratic management, the stereotyping of them as some arbitrary picture labeled "nurse" that so many people have by taking on the authoritarian role with patients, orderlies, and other people lower in the pecking order.

Old people are particularly vulnerable in this kind of situation. They often feel, and are, very much alone and unsupported. They are concerned (as are many hospital patients) that any protest against the kind of treatment they get will result in total abandonment. So they submit to taking orders without question, being treated as if they were, at best, children and, at worst, mindless. They are bathed when they could bathe themselves and "dressed up" with ribbons in their hair. Nothing could be more indicative of the antihumanistic stance of a profession committed to alleviate human suffering than the denial to old people of the dignity of their own persons.

Nurses are too often concerned solely with the observable physical needs of old people, and the tendency is to ignore everything else about them that goes to make up the human being. At least one study has indicated that, even when nurses had the psychological and social information about patients, based on nursing histories, most of them did not use this information to improve patient care.[2]

Institutions run by medical personnel—hospitals, convalescent homes—reinforce the waiting, depressing, uninvolved stance of old people. Consortiums of doctors keep the old waiting endlessly for visits—first to get an appointment, and then to wait hours after the appointed time before they can be treated. If this is done in a situation where there is some choice left to the old person, how much worse must it be in situations where there is little or no choice!

Hospitals have traditionally dealt with the multitude of details of work and patient care in the way that most of our organizations and institutions have dealt with details and large numbers of people. We always seem to resort to the principle of the assembly line, relying on interchangeability of parts and efficiency of time and motion to get the work done. Schools attempt to teach large numbers of children by pretending that each group of thirty or so is made up of individuals who are almost exactly alike. The belief is that, if one teacher teaches something at a particular rate of speed in a particular way to each unit of thirty children, they will all learn. If it becomes depressingly clear—as it inevitably does—that all thirty will *not* learn, then the system provides for (1) blaming the individuals, (2) punishing them, and, finally (3) excluding them—all in a frantic attempt to keep the units "homogeneous" and functioning efficiently.

Mass production operates in the hospital, too, and the press for efficiency in bathing and meal-serving spills over into professional-patient interaction. Consequently sitting at a patient's bedside is almost unheard of even if what that patient needs is the proximity of another human being. Putting one's arms around a patient is "unprofessional," even if what the patient needs is affectionate contact with another person. Crying with a patient who is mourning his own imminent death is reducing the competency of professional functioning, even though it is the most human thing that anyone can do.

A "good" nursing home is one that provides efficiently for meals (*not* planned by the people who eat them!) and cleanliness (Lysol smell and no clutter of personal belongings) and medical care (a series of visiting doctors and a single registered nurse). As if what made people human were all covered by food and mopped floors and regular blood-pressure checks! These things just keep people—and other animals—alive until they die.

The work of gerontologists, although not strictly part of the medical field, strongly influences the thinking of those who work with old people and have pretensions to staying *au courant* with scientific thinking. Such medical practitioners cannot help hearing about the "rolelessness" of the old with its implication that people play no part in society when they reach a certain age. The oversimplification of this concept—even in a society that pushes old people out of many of the significant roles they held when they were younger—must surely be apparent to anyone who lives intimately with an aged person. The role of loving grandmother can be either salutary or destructive, but it does exist. The role of parent takes on new forms in old age, but it does not disappear. The role of patient in old age makes a significant, if not always comfort-producing, contribution to the medical field, and the role of friend and neighbor persists. Even to strangers, the old person, by his being, poses a problem and a threat and often produces a need to respond out of fear or guilt, or remembered love.

It is, after all, only the disengaged young who speak of the rolelessness of the old—the young theorists who conceptualize scientific dicta separated from the human beings about whom they are theorizing. But things are looking up. The Administration on Aging makes some interesting proposals for research in the field, perhaps signaling a trend away from stereotyping the aged and toward a more rational approach to social assistance.[3] They first raise the question, "What definitions of aging are more suitable to program formulation than chronological age?" And they go on to suggest that other groups than the aged may have similar needs and require comparable services. Thus, native Americans, whose mortality and morbidity rates exceed those of the general population, may be victims of conditions that many old people are prey to, not because there is something inherent in the fact that they are Indians, but because something is happening to them vis-à-vis other people.

Unfortunately, the suggestions of the Division of Research and Analysis still seem, almost unconsciously, locked into the concept of special need for everyone over a certain age. Although they note that ". . . many of the problems associated with age may occur for different individuals and groups before they reach this legislatively defined age [60]," they never suggest that many of the problems associated with age may *not* occur for different individuals before the age of 70 or 80 or even 90. Although they are concerned that early retirees may need many of the aids needed by those who retire at the usual age, they really do not seem to leave much room for the hypothesis that legislation might be needed to protect a significant subpopulation unfairly forced to retire before they need to. The trend seems to be to push the designation "aged" lower rather than to focus on individual differences over the whole span of age and the spectrum of need. Perhaps those applying for research funds under the proposed guidelines, and who ultimately succeed in developing "alternatives to the chronological definition of age," will be able to recommend that chronological age not be used as a basis for relegating individuals to inappropriate patterns of life.

Another suggestion for research by the Administration on Aging is the study of successful means used by old people to cope with age-related crisis situations. The objective of such study would be to "enable organizations concerned with the elderly to develop innovative programs to assist elderly persons in utilizing their own personal coping resources more effectively."

I cannot help thinking that any such research would have to utilize a design that would select subjects at every socioeconomic level and then in some way adjust the findings for financial differences. In this way, *truly* age-related crises might be identified, rather than crises more related to inadequate income, in which the debilities of age are exacerbated.

The chances are, however, that the research done will be done on poverty-stricken or marginal people. The final recommendations made for helping people to cope will merely proliferate programs that siphon off money better given outright to the poor. In the meantime, the real age-related crises, among the poor as well as the well-to-do, remain obscured, and people are left to cope more or less effectually without assistance.

In the same publication of the Administration on Aging, studies are suggested to discover "knowledge concerning what changes occur with age which adversely affect the decision-making capabilities of older persons," with an eye to increasing "the older person's capability to make effective decisions on matters significant to their [sic] own well-being." The example given deals with the necessity for long-term care which many people—and significantly more older people—face at some time in their lives, and the decision that must be made if the outcome is to be "both satisfying and beneficial."

If I may belabor the point, the rich man who can afford nurses around the clock and a doctor on call at home is the only one who is really free to make the decision that suits him, unless there are some age-related or illness-related hindrances to effective decision making. The poor man's decision-making process may appear to be defective, but the hindrances may be only money-related. Studying only the poor man will give few data on age-related problems concerning decision making.

The Administration on Aging goes on to raise some questions that might be answered by researchers that have the potential for really raising the national consciousness concerning our society's treatment of aging people [4]:

> What national policies create unique crisis situations for the elderly?
>
> What economic and social forces enhance or diminish the social or economic capital of the elderly?
>
> What values, mores, stereotypes, and social conditions in the population at large inhibit or facilitate the achievement of freedom and independence of the elderly? Are subpopulations within the elderly affected differentially?
>
> How do the elderly respond to social and environmental conditions which impact negatively on their freedom and independence?
>
> What intervention at the national, state, and local level can reduce the negative impact of undesirable conditions which affect the elderly?

The last three questions, rewritten to be more specific to the hospital, health center, or other medical facility, can be legitimately raised and used as a foundation for changing practices within the institution.

Involving Patients in Change

No one can be more committed to effecting change than the ones being victimized by a current practice. Unfortunately, they, too, often feel powerless to do anything about a situation, or simply do not have the necessary skills. Sometimes, just helping them define a behavior, and then encouraging them to record the number of times it occurs, can set them on the path to taking a measure of control over their own lives.

One simple and relatively safe way to do this is to post two or three descriptions of behavior on a handy wall, and ask ambulatory patients to put a hash mark next to a description when they witness the behavior by a staff member. No staff member need be named, which makes the *behavior* the focus of concern rather than making a person the target for vituperation. It keeps the victimized patient anonymous, so that he need not fear retaliation (whether or not the fear is realistic). Then, at a staff meeting or a team meeting, or even at informal meetings such as lunch, the behaviors that have a number of marks can be discussed, their effects explored, and some sensitivity developed that might eliminate or reduce it.

An "affirmative action" committee would be a novel way to draw patients into the process for improving treatment of old people. Such a committee could inform each new patient of its objective. Patients could be encouraged to come to the committee with feelings or other facts concerning treatment. And regularly, a committee member could make the rounds of the patients, asking about specific behaviors that irritate, annoy, or violate individual dignity.

A graphic way of bringing home to a staff that all is not serene in a department is to distribute two cards to each patient, one card buff colored with NO written on it, and the other card red with YES written on it. Ask each patient to respond to a single question about behavior by tossing his card into a basin. There is nothing so sobering to a staff meeting than a basin full of red cards in response to such a question as: "Is there anyone on the staff who irritates you with his exaggerated politeness and constant deference to your age?"

We know from experience in trying to improve race relations in institutions and communities that without minority-group members functioning as an integral part of all deliberations, the margin for error in decision making is exceedingly large, and many of the problems are never even addressed.

In trying to improve interaction with people who are old, an institution that does not employ old people is seriously handicapped. One way to deal with this without delay (since a broad objective in eliminating ageism is the elimination of mandatory retirement at some arbitrarily fixed chronological age) is to identify a number of old people in the community and invite them to serve on a committee or to participate in staff meetings.

This really comes under the heading of involving patients, because community people are certainly potential patients. In addition they are a vital link of communication with those members of the community who are already patients. (They also help the young people they work with to increase their awareness that old people are not all alike.)

An organization such as the Gray Panthers is a good source of individuals who are alert to the need for self-determination and fate control for old people.

Two Propositions for Changing Practices

Some years ago, a small book was published that presented extremely helpful guidelines for establishing optimum interaction between majority and minority groups in organizations and communities. Although the authors never mentioned old people or relationships between age groups, the principles seem just as appropriate and useful to this problem, which more and more of us are confronting today. I have taken the liberty of adapting two of these principles so that they clearly refer to inter-age relations.[5]

1. The attitudes of new staff people coming into the institution will change more quickly and thoroughly from exposure to social interaction rather than from information and exhortation alone.

"A newcomer to a social environment or an institution where he wants to be accepted is likely to be unusually sensitive to other participants' perceptions of his behavior and to their approval and disapproval. . . . We tend to pattern our conduct after the conduct of those already in the particular situation." [6]

2. Fullest participation of old people in planning policy and program involves the participation of individuals with insight into the problems, skills in social relationships with younger people, articulateness in discussing age-relations, and the emotional poise to handle touchy subjects and situations without becoming bitter and hostile.

". . . it requires mature and friendly persons who have . . . a feeling of comfort in having psychologically worked through their own . . . feelings [about age]. Although, at first . . . representatives like this may be put in the position of dealing almost exclusively with . . . interpretation [of the problems of age], soon, if they have real leadership ability, they will take their place in the program, work for the purposes of the organization as a whole, and make their contribution accordingly." [7]

Notes

1. Mike Dolinsky, *Mind One*, Dell Publishing Co., Inc., New York, 1974.

2. Elizabeth A. Hefferin and Ruth E. Hunter, "Nursing Observation and Care Planning for the Hospitalized Aged," *The Gerontologist*, Vol. 15, No. 1, Part 1, February, 1975, pp. 57–60.

3. Division of Research and Analysis, Office of Research, Demonstrations and

Manpower Resources, Administration on Aging, Office of Human Development, Department of Health, Education, and Welfare, *Research and Development Strategy,* Fiscal Year 1975.

4. Ibid.

5. John P. Dean and Alex Rosen, *A Manual of Intergroup Relations,* University of Chicago Press, Chicago, 1955.

6. Ibid., p. 92.

7. Ibid., p. 31.

7

*attitudes and behaviors
toward aging and the aged*

identity and dignity

Independence

James Dowd, in his attempt to develop a viable theory of aging, postulates that disengagement is *not* a process mutually beneficial to the aging person and society. He sees it as a function of the deteriorating power of aging people who "are forced to exchange compliance . . . for their continued sustenance." [1]

No single observation of a facet of human interaction has ever struck me as forcefully with its validity! In the name of love, in the name of efficiency, in the interest of medical efficacy, the power of relatives, physicians, social workers, and even household employees is counterposed to the independence of the aged person. If he is to survive, he must continue to give up pieces of that independence until, long before he is dead, he is already treated as if he were incapable of making choices.

The loving son-in-law believes that his aged father-in-law should bathe every day—after a lifetime of bathing once a week. The son-in-law is meticulous. His wife really believes that cleanliness is next to godliness. And his *12-year-old* son has never had to be told to take a bath! But the old man, whose failing memory has made it impossible for him to continue to live alone in his small apartment, cannot understand what the anger, the impatience, the frowns are all about. For forty years he worked hard at his trade. He got up every morning at six, laid bricks all day, and at night came home to wash the sweat from his face and neck and arms and fall into bed. Saturday mornings he was able to sleep late—until eight. Then he would rise leisurely, bathe long and luxuriously, and dress in his only good suit, to take that six-block stroll to the cafeteria, informal meeting place of the men who did the same kind of work he did. His children, out playing in the street, felt proud as he walked by. Their father was elegant: he even tipped his hat to his eight-year-old daughter and her friends!

And now the husband of that daughter, kind enough to give him a home when his own sons and their wives would not, was implying that he was not clean enough to live in the same house with his children and grandchildren. Did he smell bad or something? He didn't even work any more—what was the need for all that bathing?

But his son-in-law insisted, so he bathed every day. But there was more to it than that. It became a game to see if he could get to bed before the younger man remembered to remind him to bathe. He would pretend absorption in the television show that everyone was watching, until it got too late for *anyone*—no matter how committed to soap and water—to insist that he bathe. And there were times when the awareness of his own powerlessness was almost overwhelming, and he ruminated with bitterness on how much it meant to a man to give up control over the small things in his life.

Another man is forced to eat breakfast at seven o'clock every morning because nobody trusts him to prepare his own simple meal after everyone else in the family has left for the day. Nor will his daughter prepare some food and leave it for him to eat when he is ready. The problem is that all his life he has been accustomed to dress, take a walk, even ride to work before he had anything to eat. He must now, at the age of 80, readjust his biological clock to suit the demands of the people who were willing to let him live out his last days in their home.

Even after a year, his daughter cannot understand why he never refers to his morning meal, and insists that the sandwich he eats at noon is his breakfast. She has shrugged it off as a minor aberration of a very old man, instead of an attempt to maintain the integrity of his individuality and a vestige of independence, even while he is forced into compliance with a routine that was never his own.

I have had some corroding personal experiences in my struggle to prevent the subjugation of my aged father. At one time, I arranged with a social agency to send us a "friendly visitor," who would help my father walk to a small neighborhood park each afternoon. Although it was strongly implied by the social worker at the agency that the visitor was carefully chosen and intensively instructed in caring for someone with my father's "problem" (occasional memory impairment, and some difficulty in walking), the social worker never observed him doing his work. She did engage in long conversations about my father and his family that rarely rose above the level of gossip. It was the sort of thing the visitor tried also to do with me on the telephone. He would try to tell me what my father had done that he shouldn't have done, what my father said that was obviously inaccurate, what my father wanted that he was not supposed to get. It was almost as if he and I were in league against (or for the care of) an old man who no longer had any propietary rights over his own life. Several times he even tried to do this when my father was present, speaking about him in the third person as if he were not even there.

One day I came home before the visitor left. "Oh," he said when he saw me. "I'll tell you now, so I won't have to call you. I won't be here tomorrow, but I'll be here on Thursday. *I'd tell him, but he'd only forget.*"

My father stood there, hearing this observation that excluded him from the conversation and carried a tone of near-contempt. For a moment I was so repelled and angry that I could do nothing but turn away. Later my father and I talked about it, and agreed that his "friendly visitor" was, at the very least, an old fool. Eventually I made it clear to the visitor that I would not engage in this kind of game with him, and I am afraid I made him rather unhappy when I made a practice of repeating verbatim to my father, in his presence, everything he told me privately. It made him unhappy, but it cured him of the obnoxious practice with me.

The social worker, on the other hand, encouraged him to continue the gossiping. It apparently gave her material to use on her incessant visits to question my poor father about things that were none of her business. And so encouraged was the friendly visitor that he, too, began to refer to my father as his "client."

The element of dependency fostered by these practices is apparent in the developing attitude of many old people toward themselves when they must rely on service of this kind. They begin to think of themselves as being troublesome to those they care about, and so many have a tendency to keep their concerns to themselves. They submit quietly to social workers and friendly visitors, relatives, and cleaning women so that their families will not think that they are too much bother. They will change the way they have lived all their lives, giving up many of their cherished idiosyncracies because a daughter-in-law, or a grandchild, or even a child of their own decides that the behavior, or the habit, or the pastime is not suitable.

If they feel like standing, they will respond to loving commands to "Sit down, Dad. You shouldn't be standing." (Maybe the son knows something the father does not.)

They will accept with equanimity the television set snapped on when they would rather just sit without the noise: "Watch television, Grandpa. Don't just sit there while we're out."

They will be sent to bed peremptorily: "It's time to sleep, Dad. You're tired." And lie in the dark for hours with eyes open, so as not to disturb the rest of the household.

There may be some justification for managing a 10-year-old's life in this way (although this is debatable, in the light of what we know about self-concept development and growth to independence), but there is really no sense to the manic rush to do unto your parent what your parent did to you. After she has nurtured you, reared you, screened your friends, and fed you oatmeal, she will probably resist the implication that she is no longer competent to continue to manage her own life.

There is a difference between being unable to live all alone and being incompetent to make the daily decisions about your personal affairs. When a person has had a serious illness and is left with a relatively debilitating chronic physical symptom, or when she has been seriously ill and is afraid to be completely alone in case there is a recurrence, it seems practical for that person to arrange to live with someone else, someone who will be able to provide the assistance needed in an emergency, or just to provide the psychological comfort that accompanies living with someone who cares. Sometimes, an individual finds that his memory is not what it once was, and he needs a reminder to take a pill or even to eat lunch.

Such debilities or feelings do not neutralize a person's need to be independent, to feel worthwhile, to keep control over his own fate. Just because the infant goes from complete dependence toward independence is no indication that the process is necessarily reversed when the individual gets old. The old person needs help in those areas where he *needs* it; it should not be forced on him in those areas where his functioning is adequate.

Actually, this precept is valid no matter what the age of the individual. The four-year-old does not need all his decisions made for him. He is quite competent to decide what he will wear to play in, or whether or not he feels like eating "another spoonful" of peas.

An adult does not become a child just because he is having difficulty in walking. An adult is not a child even if his memory is impaired and his ability to concentrate is severely limited. Perceiving him as a child and treating him like one, and then justifying it in terms of a "natural" reversal of roles that comes with the old person's dependency, is bizarre. Treating an old person like a child negates all he has learned, all he has been, all he has experienced—and, in the process, negates him as a person. To treat him as if he has forgotten many things is not the same as treating him as if he does not have anything to remember.

It often seems not to be the physical dependency of the old person as much as the almost total negation of his selfhood that results in what Robert Atchley talks about [2]:

> Many psychologists have remarked about the crisis of authority that most children encounter. This crisis may be a mere shadow in comparison to the authority crisis an older person goes through if he must become dependent on his children. Both the parent and the child resent the change, both feel guilt as a result of their resentment; and both tend to become hostile toward the source of their guilt. This kind of relationship is a vicious circle of resentment, guilt, and hostility that tends to grow increasingly worse—often to the point of a breakdown in the relationship between parent and child.

And when the son or daughter is not there, the paid nurturers take over the commands and continue the reinforcement of dependency.

I have heard a group of case workers discuss their "clients," sorting them out according to their locus of control. Thus, the "externals" are identified and efforts are made to help them shift their locus of control. (There are not many "internals," you know. The people who need help generally feel powerless to help themselves; that is their problem.)

And how does one help these people to take control of their own lives? Why, by *listing for them* the steps they can take to solve their problems! Incredible!

Just as poor people are driven into a kind of sick dependency on all the factotums of the welfare system, so old people are being coerced into a similar kind of dependency. This may prove to be a much easier job than perpetuating the dependency of the poor at this time in our history; the aged are more often handicapped by illness and physical weakness. (However, we might bear in mind Curtin's observation that old people are natural revolutionaries: they have plenty of time and nothing to lose! [3])

Social agencies are forever pointing out that there are tens of thousands of people who need help but who never ask for it. The implication is that they are the "hidden" needy, either ignorant of the facilities for help available to them or too proud to accept "charity." I think there is a third reason why people do not avail themselves of money and services provided by both public and private agencies. There is some research evidence that this is so. They simply do not want to relinquish what little control they have over their own lives. Social case workers, psychiatric social workers, law students and community lawyers, physicians and public health nurses are all eager to help. And in the process they, more often than not, assume the "client's" decision-making function in the problems of his own life.

As a race, we human beings have a propensity for knowing exactly what the other person ought to do. When that other person is in some kind of physical, mental, or financial difficulty, there is always the fleeting inference made that he brought the difficulty on himself—through neglect, ignorance, profligacy, or even hostility. Couple this idea with the self-concept of the helpers as experts in their specific area of helping, and it becomes a logical and expeditious practice to make the necessary decisions for those in trouble.

People in the helping professions usually feel that they chose their profession because they cared about people and wanted to help them. Some even profess to "love" people. Consider "loving" and "caring" in light of our operational definitions: the new lover wants to know what the beloved is thinking and feeling every second. The loving mother wants her child to epitomize *her* idea of child. The loving son is reluctant to live his own life for fear that upsetting his loving mother will make her ill. The loving father always knows what is best for his daughter.

Why, then, should the professional lover alter the customary mode of loving? As soon as the client is identified, the professional proceeds to demonstrate his loving care.

He asks questions designed to elicit intimate thoughts and feelings:

CASE WORKER: Yes, food stamps are available to help people supplement their incomes.

CLIENT: It's just temporary. My pension just isn't keeping up with inflation and rising costs.

CASE WORKER: What is your married son's income?

He makes strong suggestions for living effectively. The intimidated client rarely feels powerful enough to reject those suggestions outright:

PUBLIC HEALTH NURSE: You shouldn't have that man living here. It looks bad for your family and neighbors.

He perceives as a personal affront every attempt to circumvent rules and regulations handed down through him:

CASE WORKER: You must wait five days after applying before you can get a check.

CLIENT: But I'm desperate. There's no food in the house.

WORKER: You should have applied sooner.

CLIENT: (Revealing knowledge of information zealously kept from the public.) I was told you have a special emergency fund that you can give out without waiting.

WORKER: That's not for your kind of case. We can't just hand that out every time somebody doesn't follow the regulations. You people!

He makes decisions for clients on the basis of information that he keeps to himself:

PATIENT: Doctor, tell me the truth. Am I going to die?

PHYSICIAN: (Heartily, to patient he has just discovered has a terminal illness.) We're all going to die, some day.

PATIENT: What's the matter with me?

PHYSICIAN: Let's just concentrate on getting your treatment. Don't worry about anything else. Worry is the worst thing in the world for you. I'll see you tomorrow.

In addition to resisting the usual pressures of a bureaucracy to subjugate a clientele to its power and officiousness, the aged person must be encouraged to fight against the pressures to permit his dependency to become the reference point for all his interactions with others. The nurse who discusses clothes and politics with the 20-year-old girl in the next bed must become aware that the little old lady also has political opinions and preferences in clothes, and that she is bored to death with hearing about how devoted her children are to her. The physician must learn to include the patient, even the 80-year-old, in his discussion of symptoms and remedies and not speak only to the son or daughter, often with the parent sitting right there and being totally ignored. The white-haired man must insist, as he walks slowly and with difficulty down the street, that he not be passed over by the young person asking for signers to a consumer petition just because he cannot walk without help.

Continuity

Rosow has the following to say regarding continuity [4]:

> [P]eople are tied into their society essentially through their beliefs, the groups that they belong to, and the positions that they occupy. In general, to the extent that older people can preserve their middle age patterns in these areas, then they maintain the basis of their social integration. That is, insofar as their lives do *not* change in old age. But to the extent that their lives *do* change and they cannot maintain their earlier patterns, then their integration may be undermined. The crucial factor is not the absolute state of their associations so much as the sheer *disruption* of their previous life style, activities, and relationships. In general, the greater the change, the greater the risk of personal demoralization and alienation from society. Under these conditions, older people also ripen into significant social problems.

But so much in our culture constitutes pressure to force change on old people. The most intense change seems to occur as a function of the attitudes toward age and aging in our society. This is the change to negative concepts of self. "The available evidence suggests that as a person gets older his self-concept changes. Much of the literature indicates that these changes tend toward less positive self-views." [5] "Old people themselves tend to believe the negative stereotypes. . . ." [6]

There is little dignity in coming to the belief that one is not acceptable or worthwhile, that one is finished with the significant business of living, that one has little of importance to contribute. This is a profound disruption in the continuity of the person's essential existence and can easily contribute to the relinquishing of all independence and control over self. There is no dignity in enslavement.

And the change in self-concept with its consequent loss of dignity has implications for the total society. For all of us, the smooth flow from age to age until death, with optimum fulfillment at every age, is inevitably interrupted [7]:

> It is possible that attitudes contribute to observed maladaptive behaviors among the aged, some of which may result in premature death. Negative views of aging, life in general, and oneself may result in an old person's unwillingness or inability to seek needed health services, health care, or other types of assistance. Negative attitudes of old people may affect others in their environs, who in turn may feel free to respond negatively to old people or to ignore them completely. Negative views toward aging among the aged may reinforce negative views toward aging in the young, resulting in a feedback loop that further reinforces negative views in both young and old. The short-range effects of this feedback process may be to widen the gulf between young and old; the long-range effects may be to cause the young to dissociate themselves from their own aging. The net result of these processes may be the observed responses in the United States today of neglect and rejection of the aged and a seeming inability or unwillingness to plan for one's own old age.

There is evidence that old people in institutions have even more negative concepts of themselves than do other old people. This may also be a result of the abrupt change, being forced to give up a home and an accustomed way of life and to learn to respond to housing, eating, and associating with others within a totally new framework.

It may also be that institutionalization carries with it the very strong implication that the person is not wanted by his family and friends, that society is putting him aside, that he is being moved out of the way of the people who are getting on with the work of the world.

Disruption that occurs when one must move into a housing development for the aged may also be a blow to the self-concept, contributing to the devaluation of self. Although there is some evidence that old people in expensive retirement communities have more positive self-concepts than other old people, it is probably because their wealth gives them more of a feeling that their segregation is voluntary.

When Mormons are asked why they do not permit Black people to become ministers, they point to the proscriptions in the Bible. When you point to passages that seem to contradict those proscriptions, they tell you to speak to the Black members of the church. *They* apparently accept these limitations to their membership and agree with the implication that they are inferior to whites.

Similarly, younger people insist that old people prefer to associate with people of their own age. They periodically ask old people for their preference, and then proceed, on the basis of a significant number of responses, to advocate separate housing facilities—and whole communities —for old people.

There are factors that might be considered in evaluating the responses of those old people who say they prefer to live and associate only with other old people. If it is clear to a group of people that others stereotype them, think they are inferior, and feel uncomfortable in their presence, why should they *not* prefer to associate with "their own kind," and so avoid the slurs (both deliberate and unconscious), the rejection, and the reactive hostility precipitated in themselves? Isn't it better— more comfortable—to insist that one prefers the company of one's own group?

We have ample data in this country of what happens to rejected cohorts, such as Black people, Chicano people, native Americans, that continue to try to maintain a semblance of functioning as part of the total society. It requires superhuman ego strength to resist the assaults of the dominant group, and too many people fall by the wayside, destroyed. Ultimately, most people just give it up and live their lives apart wherever it is possible. Given the economic interdependence of victims and their persecutors, this living apart (and together) becomes a monstrously difficult task, and it, too, causes the destruction of many good people (to say nothing of the economic limitations within which too many are forced to live!). Thus to ask the victim if he prefers to live with his oppressor is an exercise in absurdity.

A second factor to be considered is the effect of being born and growing up in a society where all facets of education combine to make one accept the status quo as, not only normal, but inescapable—and even desirable. This has happened to so many women in the world. From early years, they absorb the stereotype of women that is presented to them by adults, by the communications media, by the textbooks with which they learn to read. It is not surprising that so many of them grow up believing that they are weak, emotional rather than logical, and ineffectual in the pursuits that run the world.

How far-fetched is it to think that people, reared in a world that seems to believe that 65 is the cutoff point for living, learn to believe the same thing—first about others and then about themselves? So, when asked if they prefer to live apart from the young, they may very well believe that segregation is the only right way to live. So old people, like many women, don't even realize they are being discriminated against. But, like women, the aged are beginning to marshal their forces and encourage others to engage in consciousness-raising activities. Like the women's movement, and the Black movement, the old people's movement will force the world to change.

The fight to maintain continuity can be seen in the organization of the Gray Panthers and in the self-assertion of its leader. "Adopt a life-style of outrage—a lifestyle of community," says Maggie Kuhn, and with that observation does to death the stereotype of the old as "dis-engaged." However, knowing the way prejudice works, there are many people who will rush to protest that Maggie is an exception. The refenc-ing process of perception enables them to insist that "they're all alike"—whoever *they* happen to be. If someone who obviously does not fit the stereotype is pointed out, that person is perceived as an exception: open the fence and let him out, then close the fence that encircles all of them. *They* are still all alike; the exception merely proves the rule. Since the bigot will see every person who does not fit the stereotype as an excep-tion—five exceptions, one hundred exceptions, a thousand exceptions—it is virtually useless to continue to point to those old people who are in-volved, active, concerned, and angry as evidence that the aged are no more disengaged than the majority of the national population that stays away from the polls most years.

The data we have seem to indicate that old people are interested in political affairs and try to keep informed, even more than younger people do.[8] But, because we as a people expect the aged to be more concerned with their aches and pains than they are with public affairs, many of us may be continuing to accept this expectation as we ourselves grow old. And we act the way we have always expected old people to act, thus becoming the agents for fulfilling our own stereotypic expectations.

Then along comes a Maggie Kuhn whose life-style as a child en-couraged independence and creative growth, and she says, "Live a life of community: Men and women—why not?! Young and old—why not?! Let each share what the other has!" And people suddenly discover that they have always been involved—mentally. Now they have a model who shows them they can be involved in direct and practical ways, for they know things that no one else knows and will not know until they, too, are old.

Researchers have found in measuring the mental health of old people "a degree of stability and competence rarely achieved by younger people. . . . The way in which they had learned to face and master stress had given them a distinct advantage in the toughening of their emotional fiber. It had made them as strong as the Rock of Gibraltar, able to cope with new catastrophe by drawing on seemingly limitless supply of inner resources. . . . [T]heir sense of well-being did not depend on transient changes which they recognized as a necessary part of life but rather on the fortress of strength they had built within them." [9]

To psychological strength and political interest, add freedom and time, and the old in America can be a formidable force. " 'I equate old age with freedom,' [Maggie Kuhn] said. 'Liberation from the strictures of established social structure. Freedom to pursue new objectives and new goals, try on new roles. We old people have lots of time: we don't have to work. We can rock the boat . . . and get away with it.' " [10]

But for every Maggie Kuhn who is heard there must be hundreds of vital, healthy, interested people who, just because they are old, find it virtually impossible to buck the institutions that systematically break their hold on life. One large university is a case in point. It spends thousands of dollars (all of it public money) for its on-going research on aging. It has on its faculty gerontologists, geriatrists, social workers, and others who profess interest in aging and concern for old people. Its graduate students are engaged in projects seeking to identify the needs of the aged. A man who was forced, only because of age, to retire from teaching and significant research in science education offered to continue his work at the University *without pay.* He was turned down summarily, not because there was any question of his ability or of the importance of his work, but because the administration feared "it would set a precedent." Research and erudition apparently have no connection to the application of knowledge to living, an observation that has been made before about the extensively schooled!

Frank Nelson, an English professor at the University of Hawaii, sued for the right to hold his job after the mandatory retirement age and won. " 'Old people,' he says, 'have been pushed around long enough.' "

"Frank Nelson speaks for many who are refusing to go gently into a dull and useless night of retirement. Besides taking to the courts, they are lobbying in their legislatures and forming self-help groups to win back the dignity and privileges denied them in a society that has made youth a national obsession." [11]

The professionals, I think, foster in old people and their offspring the idea that the old are either incompetent or that—competent or not— they ought to limit their expenditure of energy to meaningless tasks and routine exercises. The younger people who hold a negative view of old age may actually ". . . withdraw reinforcements for competence. Aging persons may in time come to accept the stereotypes, view themselves as deficient, and put aside intellectual performance as a personal goal. In the process, the intellectual deficit becomes a self-fulfilling prophecy." [12]

Although there are young people who see that the problems visited upon old people are their problems, too (the name of the Gray Panthers was originally the Coalition of Older and Younger Adults), I am persuaded that the movement for equality for any group must be primarily a movement of and by the people who are being discriminated against. The victims alone have the motivation to persevere through to the ultimate goal; others, although sympathetic to the suffering of the victims, are too easily persuaded to compromise. "Not so fast," "Not so far," "Only some today; more tomorrow," have too often been the words of white antiracists, the physically able who support nondiscriminatory treatment of the handicapped, and the men who believe in equal rights for women.

Younger people who learn all over again in middle age to respect their parents are in a strategic position to go beyond sympathy to empathy and become their parents' partners in the fight for life—and age—with dignity.

Notes

1. James Dowd, "Aging as Exchange: A Preface to Theory," *Journal of Gerontology*, Vol. 30, No. 5, 1975, pp. 584–594.

2. Robert C. Atchley, *The Social Forces in Later Life*, Wadsworth Publishing Co., Inc., Belmont, Calif., 1972, pp. 195–196.

3. Sharon R. Curtin, *Nobody Ever Died of Old Age*, Little, Brown and Company, Boston, 1972.

4. Irving Rosow, *Social Integration of the Aged*, The Free Press, New York, 1957, p. 9.

5. George R. Peters, "Self-Conceptions of the Aged, Age Identification, and Aging," *The Gerontologist*, Vol. 11, No. 4, Part II, Winter, 1971, pp. 69–73.

6. Vern L. Bengston, "Inter-age Perceptions and The Generation Gap," *The Gerontologist*, Vol. 11, No. 4, Part II, Winter, 1971, pp. 85–89.

7. Ruth Bennett and Judith Eckman, "Attitudes Toward Aging: A Critical Examination of Recent Literature and Implications for Future Research," in Carl Eisdorfer and M. Powell Lawton, *The Psychology of Adult Development and Aging*, American Psychological Association, Wash., D.C., 1973.

8. Matilda W. Riley and Ann Foner, *Aging and Society*, Vol. I, *An Inventory of Research Findings*, Russell Sage Foundation, New York, 1968, p. 368; Norval D. Glenn, "Aging, Voting, and Political Interest," *American Sociological Review*, Vol. 33, 1968, pp. 563–575.

9. Natalie Harris Cabot, *You Can't Count on Dying*, Houghton Mifflin Company, Boston, 1961, pp. 253–254.

10. Bill Mandel, "What Makes Maggie Kuhn Gallop—at 69?" *The Philadelphia Inquirer*, April 27, 1975, pp. 1I, 8I.

11. Carole Offir, "Old People's Revolt—At 65, Work Becomes a Four-Letter Word," *Psychology Today*, March, 1974, p. 40.

12. Paul B. Baltes and K. Warner Schaie, "The Myth of the Twilight Years," *Psychology Today*, March, 1974, pp. 35–40.

exercises in awareness
and skill development

learning to grow old

Exercise A: Values Clarification Sheet—Contact [1]

The loves of human beings have, traditionally, been parochial. We have, without questioning the circumstances or the desirability of their consequences, associated primarily with "our own kind," and forced others to do the same. To this day, in the 1970s, the most pervasive conflict, one that involves more people than almost any other current conflict, is the one that concerns the breaking down of physical barriers to interaction among different racial groups. People are beside themselves with rage, they threaten and hurt small children, they vow resistance in the name of God and motherhood—all because the law seeks to provide opportunity for their [white] children to go to school with Black children.

But there are not many who are involved in the anger and violence who admit that the issue is a racial one. Ostensibly they are opposed to busing—a fantastic euphemism in the light of the fact that millions of children are being bused to school every year, and parents fight any attempt to take this service away from them. Somehow, this cover-up of the real issue is a saving grace, a hopeful sign that people do struggle, although unconsciously, with some essential feeling of the wrongness of enforced racial separation.

We have not, of course, witnessed a similar kind of overt violence protesting the desegregation of the aged and the younger members of our society. However, violence undoubtedly rages—and guilt. But as a society, we manage to avoid any suggestion of the wholesale desegregation of the population, so our violence and guilt remain individual instead of group manifestations.

Our attitudes and behavior toward old people are part of a cultural system that our society has outgrown and that no longer serves us productively. People are living much longer today than they used to; the population of the aged is growing. Our technology developed with young people running the machines and, though our machines have changed, we have not yet changed our belief that only the young can make them work. (We once thought only young white men were able to keep the machine economy functioning. It took a world war to force us to face the fact that women and Black men were just as capable of working the factories!) We are finding it terribly difficult to break away from the magical imperative of the forty-hour five-day work week—in an economy where machines can provide for all our material needs with far fewer working hours. Women bearing children could work more efficiently for fewer hours, but we cannot seem to adapt to this idea; if a person cannot put in a "regular" work week, he is just not hired.

Similarly, old people could continue to work long after the arbitrary "retirement" age, if we would only update the anachronism that is our economy and gear it to the capacity of our technology and the reality of human psychological and material needs. "The retired of today, healthier and more vigorous than the retired of a generation ago, are seeking new roles, and this is a major challenge to our society." [2]

The problem, obviously, is a long-term educational one. Unfortunately, the people most likely to be receptive to systematic education—the children—are taught by people who have been entrusted with perpetuating the status quo. Therefore, it is as adults that we must begin a process of reeducating ourselves, opening up those areas for consideration that were closed off to us when we were children—closed off by silence, by avoidance, by the destructive behavior of the significant adults in our lives.

The first step in any process for dealing with attitudes is one that enables people to examine their values and make sure that they know exactly what they do believe. Very often we respond in specific situations by expressing an opinion or taking an action that is an ad hoc response to that situation at that point in time. If we look back on similar situations, we may very well find that our responses cannot be justified in terms of a coherent philosophy or even a practical consistency. We may say we believe in one thing, while behaving as if we believe something quite different; we may have an *intellectual* commitment to democracy, humanism, candor, and so on, but our feelings lead us into managing other people, hedging on direct questions, and acting as if we know what is good for the other fellow even if he doesn't want it.

These exercises may help you to make sure you really do know what you believe about various issues concerning old people. In addition, you may want to consider the consequences of holding each point of view before you make a decision either to change your opinion or keep it intact forever.

Following are several paragraphs relating to contact between old people and their offspring. Select the paragraph that comes closest to your own position and change the wording in it until it represents your thinking as exactly as possible. Or you may write a new position if none of the ones listed is close to the one you prefer. The idea is to get a statement about which you can say, "This is how I stand."

1. Families are a greatly overrated institution. Parents and children rarely get along well or contribute much to each other's life satisfaction, especially after children reach adulthood. Relationships are generally characterized either by constant bickering over matters that have been

the subject of controversy in the family for years, or by silence arising out of boredom and/or hostility. Grown offspring would do better to live hundreds of miles away from their parents and communicate only occasionally, mostly by letter or telephone. As for aged parents, their life span would probably be lengthened if they were free of the demands, the pressures, and the agitation that go along with close association with their children.

2. Old people have an overwhelming need to have their grown children very near them, so that they may see them, talk to them, and genrally continue the relationship started when the children were small. Without such constant, sustained contact, old people feel abandoned, lost, unable to find a viable role for themselves in their later years. It is a terrible thing to deprive old people of this desperately needed association in their final years.

3. As a society and as individuals we need the sense of continuity afforded by the contact between generations. If we cut ourselves off from our parents as they get old and we mature, we lose the benefit of their experience and we are condemned to "invent the wheel" all over again by trial and error in each generation. Continued learning from our parents is the foundation of social progress and individual effectiveness.

4. The nature of the relationship between an old person and his offspring is a function of the relationship they had with each other when they were all younger. Those who liked each other, appreciated each other's company, and profited from each others' experiences will likely want to continue the relationship even when some of them grow old. Offspring who were all taking and no giving in their relationship with their parents may find it impossible to continue their association when they must be the giving member, the one who must do the tending and nurturing. The guilty may do their "duty" by their aged parents and hate every moment they are together; or they may run from the sight of their parents hoping that distance and lack of communication will keep the guilt manageable. The key to predicting what will probably happen when a parent gets very old lies in understanding what is happening when the parent is not yet old.

Exercise B: Values Clarification Sheet— Disengagement from Work

Follow the same directions as for Exercise A. This kind of exercise need not be reserved for in-service or preservice professional courses. It might even be used as a substitute for party games—at that time during a party when the conversation turns serious.

You might make some notes on the discussion and see if there is any correlation between age and point of view: that is, do older people generally have one attitude and younger people another? If you are in the younger group, do you think your attitude is likely to change as you get older? If there is a dichotomy between the younger and the older on this issue, is it inevitable that the division will always exist? What does this bode for the future of this problem?

1. Old people should retire and leave the world to be run by young, vigorous people who still have all their faculties. Even the customary retiring age of 65 should be lowered, especially in times like these when jobs are scarce and the economy is generally in such a mess.

2. People should retire when *they* feel ready to do so. A person has the right to go on working as long as he feels that he has a contribution to make.

3. Old people have much wisdom that comes from experience. They should be given the opportunity to share their wisdom with those who are still in the decision-making positions. Of course, some process must be devised to facilitate this sharing, since people over 60 or 65 can't just go on working.

4. Just because a person lives a certain number of years does not mean that he loses his ability to function effectively in his work. Every person should be considered as an individual before a decision is made about whether or not he should retire.

5. There is enough work to do in the world if people want to do it. Volunteers are always needed, and people who have reached retirement age and no longer work at their regular jobs can do volunteer work for as long as they want or are able to.

Exercise C: How Democratic Are You?

Below is a list of questions dealing with broad values for living. Indicate in the columns provided which values are yours and which are not.

	Yes	No
1. Do you believe in the American creed of equality of opportunity for all people?		
2. Are all people entitled to equality of treatment before the law?		
3. Should laws always be obeyed?		

Yes | No

4. Is it ever all right to stand by and let another person's rights be violated?

5. Do people have a right to express their views freely?

6. Is democracy a good form of government?

7. Has anyone the right to decide that a person's life should be terminated?

8. Should there be educational mandates for the elimination of prejudice from our culture?

9. Does the government have the right, in addition to maintaining records on the vital statistics of individuals, to keep dossiers of the activities of individuals?

10. Are all people entitled to access to any government records that are kept on them and to insist on immediate deletion of errors?

11. Does an individual have the right to make a decision about how another person must live his life?

Exercise D: Checking Your Attitudes in Specific Situations

Following is a series of specific situations involving old people and their relationships with younger people. In the columns provided, answer yes or no to the question at the end of each situation, indicating how you would respond if you were the *younger person* in the situation.

Yes | No

1. A man has just been informed by his employer that he is fired as of the end of the month. He has worked at his job for fifteen years. He has been repeatedly commended for his ability, his

Yes |No

efficiency, his commitment to the work, his helpfulness to his co-workers. There is no suggestion that he is failing at any aspect of his job. He is 65 years old.

Do you believe that his employers have the right to fire him?

2. A woman turning a corner in her car injured a pedestrian. Neither the pedestrian nor the driver was, strictly speaking, in violation of the law when the accident occurred. However, the pedestrian had run out into the street so suddenly that the driver was not able to stop the car in time to prevent hitting him. As soon as the magistrate heard the story, he told the driver that she had no business to be driving and that he was going to recommend that her license be revoked. The driver is 70 years old.

Do you think the magistrate has the right to have her license revoked?

3. Ms. Jean Staser and Mr. Robert Crale are living together as man and wife without benefit of clergy. Not only are they violating the laws of their church, but they are also in violation of the laws of the state; the law does not recognize common-law marriage. In addition, the laws against adultery and fornication are clear and, at the moment very much in the consciousness of the people, because there is a concerted movement to reverse what is feared to be a growing trend against formal marriage.

Jean and Robert continue to resist the pressure of the people they know to formalize their marriage. They insist that the only way they can survive is to pool their financial resources. Getting married would mean that their income would immediately be reduced. (They are obviously also breaking the *spirit* of the federal law, even if they are abiding by the letter of the law.)

Jean and Robert are both collecting Social Security retirement benefits.

Do you believe that Jean and Robert have the right to break the law if they think it is in their best interests, and it does not violate the rights of anyone else?

4. Evelyn Price is a registered nurse in a home that caters to old people. Although it is called a convalescent home, it houses people who are not recovering from any specific illness: they just live there.

Although Ms. Price has grave doubts about many of the practices of the staff, she particularly objects to what is being done to

Mr. Brown. He gets around by himself, even though he does so slowly and with a little difficulty. During the day nobody interferes with him as he walks from room to room—to the bathroom, to the recreation room, etc.—without assistance.

At night, however, he has been repeatedly admonished that he is not to go to the bathroom. He must first take great care not to drink any liquids too late in the evening, and he must use the bathroom before he goes to bed. In the event that he *absolutely must* use the bathroom in the middle of the night, he is instructed to wait until the night attendant looks in, and ask for a bedpan. This restriction of his freedom is making him miserable. He feels that he is being forced into an invalid role when he still is able to care for his own needs.

Evelyn Price really believes that Mr. Brown's rights are being violated. She does not believe that, for the sake of expediency or the questionable validity of the belief that it is being done "for his own good," the home administrators have the right to restrict his freedom in this way.

Mr. Brown has been placed in the home by his grown children, who rarely come to see him or attempt to keep in touch with him in other ways. He himself feels too old and feeble to take a strong stand for his rights—or just get up and go to live someplace else.

Do you think that Evelyn Price should stay out of the matter? Since she works only during the day, do you believe that she should not get involved?

5. John Case's income is insufficient for him to live comfortably, and he is unable to find work suited to his ability. Some time ago, his son and daughter-in-law offered him the opportunity to live in a downstairs room in their house and share meals and the use of the living room with them and their two children. In exchange, he has turned over most of his small income to his daughter-in-law, knowing very well that it doesn't begin to reimburse her for the comfort she provides for him in her home. He knows that he would really be in trouble if he did not have his family to depend on. He has friends his own age who have forgotten the taste of meat, and who live in such bad conditions that their health is in serious jeopardy. He is very grateful.

He is also forever mindful that he is completely dependent on the continued goodwill of his son and daughter-in-law. This constant awareness of dependency is sharpened by the real differences in political belief between him and his family. He has been something of a radical all his life, and his daughter-in-law, particularly, is extremely conservative in her perception of social issues and political candidates. Privately, John Case thinks some of her views approach totalitarianism and bigotry. She has made it clear that she will not tolerate "radical talk" in her house and in front of her friends, especially not with her children.

Do you agree with the daughter-in-law that she has a right to demand that in her house John Case should keep his unacceptable ideas to himself?

6. Twenty-six people live in a house run by a proprietor and six employees. The proprietor decides what the twenty-six people should have for their meals and when those meals should be served. The woman who does the general cleaning takes it upon herself to reprimand the people when she thinks they are not as neat and clean as they should be. The decision has been made—again by the proprietor—that everyone should be in bed, with lights out, by 10 o'clock. Visitors may visit only in the recreation room or, in warm weather, on the porch. The residents may come and go as they please, but they must sign in and out, and they may not leave if the proprietor decides the weather or the time or anything else is not appropriate. It is the proprietor who decides when someone needs a doctor (although the residents are responsible for their own medical costs). Generally, the proprietor seems to have a role similar to the one of head of an orphanage. The proprietor maintains that, since the house belongs to her, and since she is paid to provide comfort for the residents, she is obliged to take what measures are necessary to fulfill her responsibility. She insists that the residents don't want the bother of making the decisions. And, anyhow, most of them, because of their age, are not capable of making the best decisions.

Do you agree that the proprietor has the right and the responsibility to run her house this way?

7. Jean Hilton is very active in a movement to get younger people to sign statements saying that, should they ever be unable to speak for themselves and are being kept alive only by machinery, the medical personnel have permission to discontinue these extraordinary measures and permit life to end.

Jean believes that the machines that breathe for a person and pump his blood are an obscenity, that they rob the individual of his final dignity and that there is no justification for prolonging this travesty of life, a life without thinking or feeling or any power of control over one's self.

Jean's mother suffered a stroke when she was 65. For eight

months she lay in a coma, with her body functions managed by the machines. All the money they had in the world was spent for hospital bills, and Jean went into debt, which it will take a long time to repay, while the doctors kept telling her that there was no hope that her mother would ever come out of it.

Part of what drives Jean Hilton is the fear of being old. She is profoundly convinced that when a person can no longer do his life's work, there is no point in continuing to exist. She herself is a registered nurse, and she dreads the thought of being forced to retire. She is also, now at the age of 40, aware of a growing desperation as she views the inexorable signs of aging in her mirror.

If the signers of those legal permissions (living wills) ever grow to significant numbers and the law is changed to eliminate the risk that medical people run by acceding to those permissions, Jean would like to see committees set up to make the final decisions on individual cases. She would be the first to volunteer to sit on such a committee.

Do you believe that people should be encouraged to sign the permissions, that the law should be changed to protect the decision makers, and that committees of qualified persons should be set up to make the decisions?

8. Mrs. Wolfe is a third-grade teacher in the public school system. She is assigned to teach the children confined to the pediatric wing of General Hospital. She is teaching a unit on "People of Our World" as a part of the curriculum in social studies. She starts out by asking the children, who range in age from five to thirteen, "What do you want to know about old people?"

As the children give their responses, she writes down what they say with a felt pen on a large piece of newsprint. When the responses stop coming, she promises to give them a chance to get answers to all the questions they have raised. She also promises to give each child a copy of all the responses so that they may make decisions about the order in which they deal with the responses.

The next time she comes to the ward, she distributes the copies of the responses and prepares to discuss with the children how they wish to begin their study of old people. Mrs. Smith, an 80-year-old woman who is a patient in the hospital and a friend of Mrs. Wolfe's, has come to sit in on the lesson.

A parent comes in as Mrs. Smith, the teacher, and the children are sitting together at the low round table in the room. She listens for a few moments and then leaves. When Mrs. Wolfe finishes teaching for the morning, she is waylaid in the corridor

Yes | No

by the parent, who by now is apparently very disturbed.

"I think it's terrible what you're teaching those children!" she almost shouts.

Mrs. Wolfe is bewildered. "I don't understand," she says. "What are you talking about?"

"I saw some of those things on the papers you gave them. Things like, 'I know an old witch,' and 'There's a crazy old man on my block. He scares all the children.' That's terrible!"

"But I'm not teaching the children those things; those are the things *they* said," Mrs. Wolfe protests.

"Children should be taught to be loving! They shouldn't be permitted to say things like that!"

"I agree with you. Children should be loving. But if I don't know how they feel, how can I help them learn to be different?"

"What are you trying to do, make them out to be little monsters? You're suposed to be the teacher; why don't you tell them what they're supposed to know instead of asking them. They don't know about these things. They don't know *what* they want!"

"I think," Mrs. Wolfe says gently, "that they will learn better if I provide opportunities for them to find out for themselves. I have all kinds of stories and films and other things to help them add to their experience."

But the parent's position just continues to harden: "I don't know why you're teaching them about old people, anyhow! You're supposed to teach them reading and writing and arithmetic. If they have to learn about old people, they'll learn at home!"

Do you believe that children should be taught in school to deal with the problems of prejudice and discrimination?

9. A group of scientists on the faculty of City University have just received a \$350,000 grant from the federal government to conduct research on aging. The group is made up of a biologist, a gerontologist, a psychometrist, a psychiatrist, a geriatrics specialist, and a social worker.

The research design involves using a population of old people served by several social agencies. The social workers who make personal contact with the old people will be instructed to ask certain questions of their clients for purposes of the study, without being explicit about what those purposes are.

Although the old people come to the social agencies for a variety of reasons, they will all be asked a number of specific questions designed to collect information about their political knowledge, attitudes, and involvement. The questions are asked in such a way that they sound like casual conversation, and, although the clients are told—also casually—that a study is in progress, they

Yes | No

really do not know that these questions and their responses are part of the study.

One of the provisions of the federal grant is that all information gathered by the researchers be made a part of the records of the old people for the files of a department of the federal government.

Do you believe that scientists, with the assistance of the government, have the right to gather information about individuals and keep it on file for purposes of scientific research?

10. When the study just discussed (in question 9) has been over for a year, some of the clients accidentally discover its purposes, and they learn that information about them has been computerized and is stored in the files of the federal government. A group of them decide to send a delegation to the local federal building and ask to see what is in their files. The local official receives them courteously, but he cannot hide his amusement at their request.

"Really," he protests gently, "You shouldn't be so disturbed. What do you think the government is planning to do to you? Why don't you all stop worrying about this and go home? You're perfectly safe, you know. Your government only wants to do its best for you."

Do you think the clients of the social agency have the right to demand that they see their files, and to demand also that certain things be removed?

11. Ellen Fielding, John Crouse, James Fuller, Harold Court, Sylvia Service, Rose Franks, and her sister Evelyn all live in an apartment house in the city. They are all friends and range in age from 70 to 76. Because they live on the fixed income of Social Security and some small pensions, their social activity is very limited. They like to go to the movies, but the movie theatres are just a little too far for some of them to walk to. The buses are very inconvenient, because some of them cannot take that first step up, and it is embarrassing to have strangers pulling and pushing them every time they want to get on or off the bus. The cost of taxis is prohibitive.

The friends also like to go to the theatre and the opera, and, occasionally, to a restaurant, but the tickets are much too expensive and food prices in restaurants are very high for people on limited incomes.

Some of them are avid readers, and they even like to read aloud to the others sometimes. Going to the local library presents

Yes | No

almost as many difficulties as going anywhere else, because it is so far.

Just recently, a social service agency has obtained some local and federal money and has opened a senior citizens center near the apartment house where the group lives. The center is asking people to come in and play cards, which the friends detest. There are exercise classes, which are of no interest at all to *anyone* they know. There are lectures on diet and Social Security that offer information readily available in the daily newspapers, and an occasional picnic outing, with all the fuss and discomfort that are a part of picnics.

The center is used by a few people who sometimes wander in and usually wander out again after a little while. Five or six people participate enthusiastically in the program, but most of the people in the area really do not want this kind of program. Mostly, they don't want to participate in prescribed activities with strangers.

The group of friends, talking one day over coffee, come to the conclusion that sooner or later they will be compelled to use the center because they cannot afford to do what they would really like to do. They wonder why, instead of a center run by people who decide how you should spend your time, the government cannot just divide the money among those with limited income and trust them to use that money in the way that adds to their own comfort and enjoyment. Rich people are never programmed, they think. Why do government and social workers think they are needed to program poor people?

Do you think the government should pay young people to develop social and leisure time programs for older people?

Exercise E: An Exercise in Empathy

Now, using the items in Exercise D, indicate how you would respond if you were an old person in the situation.

Exercise F: How Consistent Are You in Your Values and Attitudes?

Compare your responses in Exercises C and D and try to determine if there are any inconsistencies between your professed values and your attitude in specific situations. Indicate, also, those areas where your attitudes accurately reflect your values. Now look at the column where you checked your attitude as an old person. Are you maintaining some consistency here, or do you believe that your attitudes and values will change when you get old?

Check your responses in Exercises C, D, and E with the chart that follows.

Comparison Sheet for Exercises C, D, and E: Responses That Score for Democracy

Item	Exercise C	Exercise D	Execise E
1	Yes	No	No
2	Yes	No	No
3	Yes	Yes	Yes
4	Yes	No	No
5	Yes	No	No
6	Yes	No	No
7	Yes	No	No
8	Yes	Yes	Yes
9	Yes	Yes	Yes
10	Yes	Yes	Yes
11	Yes	No	No

Give yourself 3 points for each response that matches the one in this chart. Add 1 point to your total to permit a perfect score of 100. If you got 100, you are the perfect democrat—too good to be true.

Each time you discover an inconsistency between D and F, deduct 6 more points as a special penalty for believing that a person's basic values change just because he gets old.

Discussion

EXERCISE A: Students discussing the four points of view in this exercise often experience great discomfort. On the one hand, they hold what they believe are cultural and humanistic values on the sanctity of the family, the concern for the weak and elderly, the love of children for their fathers and mothers. On the other hand, they inevitably harbor feelings that seem to be at great variance with these values. They sometimes hate their parents, they are often in profound disagreement with their views. If they live with their parents, they often wish they did not. If they have left the family home, they often feel guilty, because their parents are not happy about the separation.

Rarely, one finds a young person who loves and respects her parents, enjoys and profits from her association with them, and at the same time has made a life for herself away from them, without recriminations or guilt.

Older adults and their aged parents show similar patterns of conflict and stress. If they live together, there is usually more conflict between them than when they do not. Most parents, when they live apart from their grown children, feel that they don't see them often enough. Grown children feel some guilt about not seeing their parents more often. Generally, however, both parents and grown children prefer to live in separate households.

Specifically, in examining the first point of view, that when grown children and aged parents stay away from each other they are doing each other a favor, most adult discussants start out with nervous laughter. Then they begin to protest that they do not feel this way at all, that they love their parents and get along well with them, that they have very close-knit families and generally good relations. As the discussion proceeds, they begin to tell anecdotes illustrating the accuracy of the statement.

One woman confessed that she really had never liked some of her father's behaviors, and now that she was an adult, she resented having to be exposed to them. His vulgar table manners, his dirty fingernails, the clothes he wore until they fell off his back in rags, even though he could afford new clothes. As soon as she saw him, it was like a reflex response —she began to nag him about these things. Naturally he disliked the nagging, but even more, he was hurt at the clear implication that his daughter disapproved of him and was ashamed of him. The bickering invariably ended with cold silence on both sides, relief when they parted, and self-recrimination on the woman's part for "being so mean" to her father.

At least one recent researcher indicates that parents and grown children have a relatively high self-evaluation of "family cohesion" (74 percent of the parents and 60 percent of the adult children say they form a "close family group"), yet only 40 percent of the parents and 24 percent of the children want a good deal more interaction with each other.[3]

Rosenmayr suggests that, to get a more accurate picture of parent-sibling relationships, what is needed is study of the communicative content of the interaction between the generations. "What, for example, is the degree of interest that adult children have in talking to their parents? What are topics of common interest in various educational and occupational groups? How strong is the influence of overt value positions of the parents on their adult children, and in what areas of decision-making?"[4]

Many younger people who discussed the second point of view seem bent on proving—probably to themselves—that their elderly parents are quite happy living their own lives. One man described in detail the fine Home his father lived in, where church volunteers increased the ratio of worker to patient to a startling three to one.

Another man told about how content his father was, living in a retirement hotel, having his meals prepared, his friends around him. He understood that his children were busy and had their own lives to live. He didn't expect frequent visits from them; as long as he knew they were well and happy, he was satisfied.

Whatever research evidence we have indicates that neither older parents nor children, in countries and cultures that differ widely, want to live together.[5] However, "There is some evidence that parent–child relations are not fully reciprocal, inasmuch as aged parents seem more attached to their children than vice versa. Old people, far more frequently than younger ones, consider that they see too little of their families." [6]

Perhaps, the answer lies in what happens to old people in contemporary life, during this transition period in which we find ourselves, in which there are many more old people who are faced with making a life for themselves in a society that provides few guidelines and little help for them.[7]

If old people were permitted to continue the tenor of their lives with some reasonable approximation to the pattern they had chosen for themselves in their earlier years, they would feel less need to invest themselves so totally in their parent role in later years. Most young parents, because they have so many other things to do, so many other meaningful roles to play, feel nothing but relief when they have the opportunity to step out of their parent roles for periods of time. If there is a sense of powerlessness, and nothing else to do, all life is focused on the waiting for the children who are no longer children.

Point of view number 3 makes many people smile. I think that, as a society, we have never really learned how to learn from the experiences of our elders. It may have something to do with the quality of our interaction, first at home and then in school. Teachers, particularly, encourage a rejecting scepticism of most of what they have to offer. They too often insist that (1) pupils don't know what's good for them; (2) the way to teach is to tell them what you want them to know; (3) if you don't take a firm, hard line, pupils will take advantage of you and the situation; and (4) youngsters don't really want to learn, you must force them to do so. The result of such a philosophy of teaching is that young people begin to resist out of hand everything older people stand for. The "don't trust anyone over 30" is a reactive prejudice, a reaction to the obvious distrust that older people feel for youngsters.

When it becomes clear that so much of what teachers teach really is worthless, has little or no relevance to the world or what needs to be done, stifles creativity and thereby actually impedes progress in solving critical problems, then the original resistance is reinforced.

The stereotype of old people in our society as having nothing to offer, added to the general rejection of older people by the young, makes old people the victims of the young. The young, growing into middle age, retain the stereotype, and the suggestion that they need the life wisdom of the old becomes merely laughable.

The fourth point of view seems to be consistent with some of the research findings in the field, and also with the observation here that relationships between children and adults mitigate against openness, trust, and acceptance. "Three-generation dwelling under one roof is almost as common as it ever was. But whereas it previously took the form of a younger family living in the grandfather's large home, now it is likely to be the case of a widowed grandmother added to a young family's limited quarters." [8]

"Conflict is likely to be greatest when economic reasons force the old and the young together and when traditions of subordination of the young are loosened." [9]

The facile assumption is that the stresses of economic problems cause the conflict. Although one must not minimize the disruption that can be caused because of too little money, more significance I think, shows in the phrase, "traditions of subordination of the young. . . ." This is the key to a pattern of relationship that is instituted by parents when children are too small and too powerless to resist. The years of frustration and unresolved hostility result in the resentment of adults who must live once again with aged parents. Conflict is inevitable.

However, researchers see mainly the fact that offspring are helping their parents, are taking them into their homes. Then they listen to both aged parents and offspring assert that they are satisfied with the amount of help given and received. "Several data have shown that the degree of help desired by the elderly equaled the amount the young generation was willing to give and actually gave. . . . Most studies have taken help patterns as the core of data for the statement of established positive interaction patterns between the generations. . . ." [10]

More work needs to be done on the analysis of the *quality* of the interaction in the new family unit. It would be even more useful to conduct longitudinal studies of the quality of interaction, following the family unit from marriage through the rearing of children, on to the time when the parent comes to live with the adult child.

EXERCISE B: Consider again your belief that old people's attitudes are consistently different from those of young people.

Maggie Kuhn, the best-known Gray Panther, may not be typical of old people, but she can be studied as evidence that basic attitudes and values in old age are merely kept with the passing years. It would appear that Ms. Kuhn's values and attitudes are energetically acted upon—this is what distinguishes her from most old people. She is someone who has not permitted people to foist their expectations on her and to make her conform to their stereotype of the aged.

"Maggie Kuhn has been concerned about social issues all her life." [11] She was born to a woman who also was concerned, so her values and attitudes were part of her childhood—as is the case with most of us. "[H]er mother traveled to Buffalo from Memphis when Maggie was born in 1905 to avoid having her baby in the South. Mrs. Kuhn couldn't stand the segregated policies then current in the South."

She was a radical as a girl and she is a radical today. But audiences, listening to her, wonder that an old person can be a radical. But why should she be anything else? Why would her view of the world and people change much between the age of 50 and 60—or 40 and 50? No, it is not conceivable that a humanist, a believer in equality, an antiracist at 20 can just naturally evolve into an authoritarian and a bigot at the age of 70.

EXERCISE C—SITUATION 1: The question we have to ask ourselves is: "How is retirement different from firing?" One gets a rush of responses, ranging all the way from: "A person has a *right* to retire after working for most of his life" to "You've got to move the old people out and give the young people a chance at the jobs." In all of them, however, the core of the opinion is stereotyping; each person is not considered as an individual, with individual needs and capabilities. The picture in the mind is of a *group, all* of whom want to retire, *all* of whom are senile, or feeble. ("All," for stereotypers, saves the day for apparent rationality by making "exceptions.") Of course, *all* old people are not senile; there *are* exceptions. The net effect, however, is to treat all of them as if they were senile.

The case for moving old people out of work to make room for the young is, from the humanistic as well as the legal point of view, on very shaky ground. How can it be acceptable to destroy one group of human beings for the benefit of another group of human beings? The argument once ran that the African slaves were happy, since they were so cherished and cared for; now the analogous argument has it that old people want to "rest," or, somewhat more scientifically, that it is "natural" for them to disengage themselves from many of the activities that were once so important to them.

Actually, there is no doubt that there is a part of the population that is quite happy to be rid of its "life's work." When that work was entered upon in youth that provided no viable alternatives; when that work is, at best, dull and, at worst, destructive of mind and body; when enthusiasm and creativity were systematically dampened in school, so that the young person believed he could do nothing but what he finally began to do, then it is understandable that he looks forward to retirement with eagerness, and reaches it with a sigh of relief.

For those who do work that fulfills them in one way or another, leaving that work is a beginning of dying. We have deluded ourselves into believing that young men must periodically go to war and die so that others may continue to live in their accustomed style. Are we also saying that young people cannot productively continue the course of their lives unless old people die?

Old people vote. As a group they can have clout, if they vote in their own interests. Sharon Curtin says that the aged are natural revolutionaries: they have plenty of time and nothing to lose! [12] They can resist this violation of their human right to continue to live. Are the laws that mandate equality of opportunity like our "All men are created equal"? That one really meant, "All *white* men. . . ."

SITUATION 2: In a traffic case where fault is not clear cut, there is usually some attempt at mediation. The outright assumption that the fault lies in the physical and/or mental condition of the driver is clearly a violation of the individual's right to freedom from discrimination, for no such assumption would have been made if the driver presented the same physical and mental appearance but had fewer wrinkles and no gray hair.

The discussants of this situation, like the judge, also go immediately to the age of the driver, implying, by their observations and the questions they ask, that they already hold some opinions on the advisability of permitting such a person to drive. As soon as they hear that the driver is 70 years old, they say, "Well, reflexes *do* slow down after a certain age." Slow down from what? I may ask. This particular person's reflexes may always have been so quick and keen that, even if age had slowed them, she could still be far more qualified to drive than are many 30-year-olds. They ask, "What about her eyesight?" Would they ask that if she were 25? Yet one-fourth of 25-year-olds need glasses, and many of them don't wear the glasses they need.

Finally, then, the discussion gets to the critical point. "Really," someone says, "Should 70-year-olds be permitted to drive? Oh—more for their *own* safety than for the safety of others! I have nothing against old people: I just want to protect them from themselves!"

SITUATION 3: There seems to be some ambivalence in the attitudes toward the people in situation number 3. Even young people who demand for their own age groups the right to live together without marriage often feel some repulsion at the idea that their grandparents might do the same thing.

Apparently, the fact that the law is being violated is not the deciding factor in most people's assertion that Jean and Robert should not live together without benefit of clergy. A number of people see the necessity for ignoring archaic law and even breaking discriminatory law as a protest and as a first step toward getting those laws changed, as when people prevent access to workers on a building site where skilled Black workers are not hired.

A few are concerned with the moral aspects—that it is sinful for a man and woman to live together in this way. Another few seem to agree but are reluctant to say so; their early upbringing comes into conflict with their intellectual rejection of religious scruples.

Most of the discussants, however, relate their attitudes to a sense of the fitness of things. These two old people disturb their sense of decorum. Old people just should not behave this way: it isn't right. They should not be ruffling the waters, rocking the boat. They should be quiet, and conventional, modeling the old virtues. It is all right for them to be crotchety and disagreeable—that comfortably confirms the stereotype of old people—but they must not step out of the stereotypic role by raising serious legal and moral questions.

SITUATION 4: All discussants respond to question 4 in Exercise B with a categorical and resounding "No!" It is, simply and unarguably, *wrong* to permit the strong, the ruthless, the criminal to take advantage of the weak and vulnerable. After all, isn't that what our system of law is all about—that the powerless have the right to expect they will be protected from the depredations of the powerful?

As the discussion proceeds, however, it becomes increasingly clear that the commitment to personal responsibility for protecting the rights of everybody is hedged about with many qualifications. There are the police—it's their job to deal with violence. There are agencies—it's their job to investigate and intervene.

Most people say they would certainly take a step—albeit a timid one—to inform the appropriate agency if they saw someone being taken advantage of. But what agency would undertake to intervene on behalf of a patient who is being forced to use a bedpan? And is it really such a dreadful violation that one should cause anger and hostility on the job? There really is nothing so terrible about using a bedpan at night. It's probably safer for Mr. Brown than getting off the bed and wandering around in the dimly lighted corridor. The administrators have only his best interests at heart. The old man is just being stubborn—so characteristic of old people.

Why make a fuss about nothing?!

SITUATION 5: Freedom of speech is a value greatly treasured in the United States. Too often, however, it seems treasured only in the abstract, as if the children now grown are recalling their fourth-grade social studies lessons learned by heart. Adults even repeat airily the aphorism, "I may disagree with what you say, but I will defend with my life your right to say it."

But in a group of thirty-five professionals, ten will say that some form of censorship is necessary, although they invariably disclaim any liking for censorship. (Of course, when it comes to censoring what children see and hear and even talk about, the percentage of those who believe in censorship goes up precipitously. I cannot help remembering how alarmed a number of teachers, parents, and a principal became when I asked a group of Black children, "What do you want to know about white people?" and the children told me what they wanted to know. The adults insisted that the children didn't think about white people, saw no differences between races, and didn't want to know anything about this. The children's responses, of course, gave the lie to all this. But the point is that the children's right to express wishes and opinions was being arbitrarily limited—by people who were teaching these same children that freedom of speech is guaranteed to everyone by the Constitution.)

John Case came to live with his family. His payment for this was made partly in money and partly with his freedom. There was never any question of his being at home—it was clear that he was living in someone else's home, and that he would have to limit his speaking to those topics and those viewpoints that were approved by the owner.

SITUATION 6: Just as most adults believe in freedom of speech, so most maintain that democracy is the best form of government, or, at least, the best that human beings have ever been able to devise. Despite this belief, however, there are few situations in which people are permitted to function democratically. Always those in charge have reasons why democracy is not feasible in this particular situation. In schools, the children are too young for democracy. In hospitals, the patients don't know enough about medicine to participate in the decision making. (Is this also true of the nurses?) The armed services are *proudly* undemocratic. The police department takes its pattern from them. The factory and the office are run by people who are "entitled" to run them, the owners or their designated representatives.

Where, in the everyday intimacies of life, in the living that has meaning for us, do we give evidence that we believe in democracy? It is no wonder that our political forms are just that—forms. Most people do not even vote regularly, and the pervasive feeling is one of powerlessness. "The politicians run the country; there's nothing the ordinary citizen can do to influence them."

If this is the pattern in our society, the question may well be asked, Why bother to change it in a house for old people? If *anyone* would be reluctant to take on the responsibilities that accompany democratic involvement, it would be old people, who are probably quite content to spend their remaining years free from the bother and fuss that comes with involvement.

Undoubtedly, there are some individuals who are content to fit into a situation where all decisions are made for them. Generally, however, we are not so content to sit back and permit others to regulate our personal habits. Although we feel at the mercy of institutions, and usually accept what is "customary," we are unusual indeed if, as adults, we are accepting of authoritarian determination of our time for sleeping, what we eat, and whether or not we feel uncomfortable enough to need the services of a physician. These kinds of decisions are made for children: they are not generally made for adults, except older adults. The assumption is—*not* based on evaluation of the people involved—that older adults cannot and/or prefer not to make their own decisions.

SITUATION 7: One way of coming to a clear and rational point of view on the whole matter of controlling the time of death is to examine the qualifications of the persons who are ready to assume responsibility for doing the controlling. In the case of Jean Hilton, we have a woman to whom a chosen profession is the most important thing in life. Her criterion for evaluating the worth of a person's existence is the ability to continue to work at what one has done all his adult life. Without that work, life's meaning is gone.

When Jean looks at old people, she sees herself becoming one, and it frightens her. She wants to continue to be hard-working, independent, healthy, and unwrinkled, and if she cannot be all those things, she does not want to live. Old people have no reason for living.

If we carry the case of Jean to its logical conclusion, we may be confronted with someone who not only wants to end the nonlife existence of a person whose only sign of life is an abnormal brain pattern, but with someone who sees old age generally as nonlife and may, conceivably, one day advocate ending all lives at the age of 65. Absurd? Perhaps. But a logical absurdity that needs to be taken seriously in the light of continuing population growth and increasing takeover of work by machines. In the foreseeable future (although, perhaps, not in a thousand years) competition for jobs will become more desperate and distribution of goods will become even less efficient than it is now, and there will inevitably be people who, in the light of the unsolved problems, will be viewed as contributing to the insolubility, and therefore as expendable.

If a Jean Hilton is rejected as a judge of who is to live and who is to be permitted to die, then perhaps a John Smith or a Mary Jones will be elected or appointed. John Smith thinks Black people are inherently inferior to whites. He thinks Jews are reprehensible and Catholics not to be trusted. Foreigners have no place in our culture unless and until they shed every vestige of their foreignness, and women have their place in the home and should be kept there.

When John Smith serves on a jury, as long as capital punishment has been abolished, he will be unable to send someone to his death because that person belongs to a group Smith views as culpable, suspicious, or out of place. Will we care enough to keep him from taking part in other life-and-death decisions?

Mary Jones is a physician. She is an extraordinarily skillful surgeon and is respected for her ability by colleagues. She does not spend much time with patients, except for the first consulting visit, where she corroborates the primary physician's tentative diagnosis, and the postoperative check. Unless there are complications that require further surgical intervention, she does not see the patient, relying instead on the reports of the surgical residents. At no time does she engage in conversation with the patient that does not relate directly to the surgery. She will ask a specific question about pain and motion, she will give an order, and that is the extent of patient-surgeon communication.

One almost gets the feeling, as one follows Dr. Jones on her rounds, that she does not even *see* patients. What she sees are more-or-less defective machines that are undergoing repair or consigned to the scrap heap. Make no mistake about it—Dr. Jones brings considerable skill and vast knowledge to her treatment of patients, and she does everything she can to make them well. But she has no illusions about the limitations of medicine, and, once she decides that nothing more can be done, she will spend not a moment longer with the patient or anyone who has contact with him.

It is difficult to know how Mary Jones feels about the life of a man who has about three months more to live. He can no longer work, he is confined to bed, he needs continuing care, but nothing that is done can materially change the quality of his life or prolong it. Dr. Jones doesn't know, and apparently doesn't care to know, that the patient is living out his last weeks with interest and love. He is preparing for his family's future, he is learning to communicate with his wife and children in more profoundly loving ways, and he is dying with a sense of fulfillment that lends meaning to his bereavement.

Dr. Jones knows only that the man cannot be helped by her medical/surgical skill. He no longer exists for her. Is she the person—chosen to make a decision because of the respect people have for her professional expertise—is she the one who should have the power to decide when a life has become a nonlife?

SITUATION 8: Almost everybody believes that he is not prejudiced. Almost everybody also believes that children should be reared to believe that all people are equal and deserve equal treatment. There are state guides that strongly suggest—if they do not mandate—that children should be taught about different racial, religious, and nationality groups in ways that will encourage understanding and acceptance of all people.

I know of no department of education that publishes guidelines for teaching children to understand and accept old people.

Is there an implicit assumption that children just naturally accept old people, and so no special education is necessary? If that is really so, how does it happen that adults—those children grown—so consistently stereotype, isolate, and neglect old people in our society?

Or is it rather that adults, themselves fearful of aging and dying, respond with anxiety and resistance to any attempt to expose their children to the subject?

And who speaks for the children? Are they condemned to have their lives circumscribed by the limitations of the adults around them, or are they entitled to learn everything there is to learn, even if their parents and teachers have never learned some things? Do parents *own* their children and so have the right, because they have the power, to limit the extent of their knowledge? Or do children have rights of their own because they are sentient human beings—even before they can make decisions and hold value positions?

No parent has the right to deprive a child of food and so make him die. Why, then, do so many people believe that a parent has the right to deprive a child of information—intellectual sustenance—and so make a part of him never come alive at all? Do parents own only parts of the child, such as his brain, and not other parts?

Some maintain that when the child is adult and so free of his parents and teachers, he may then make his own decisions about what to learn and what to value. Sadly, this rarely works. The child deprived of knowledge and indoctrinated with values is never really able to arrive at opinions freely; every issue, every experience is perceived in the light of what he has already learned—or been kept from learning. As the years go on, his experiences merely reinforce his early teachings. Few people have the acuity of vision and the self-awareness to free themselves from prejudices and values learned from parents and teachers, or to free themselves to accumulate the kind of information that will permit them to view the world in new ways.

Historically, schools have been entrusted with something called the "socialization" of the child. It is odd how, as soon as the school attempts to define socialization by touching on alienated groups of people, the cry goes up that this is best left for the home to do. So teachers breathe a sigh of relief, and parents close tight the almost-opened doors, on the aged, the dying; Black people, Puerto Rican people, Chicanos; the physically handicapped (or, as some say, physically *inconvenienced*) and the mentally handicapped. Everyone wants his children to be "loving," but one must love only those groups on the approved list, and only *seem* to love those that our mores say *should be* loved.

SITUATION 9: There have always been people who warned against the growing propensity of governments to gather information on the activities of private citizens. Such information, ready to hand, can easily be used to intimidate and coerce, so that, while we sit placidly and contemplate our democracy, democratic processes are being secretly subverted.

Since Watergate, even more of us are sensitive to the inroads being made on our privacy by zealots who fear dissension, zealots who thrive on the ability to predict outcomes of events, zealots who love the orderliness of each human being with a number and a file of his own.

In our own zeal to become a part of the frenzy of discovery and innovation, we are often seduced by the label "research" to permit the further erosion of our privacy.

In the name of research, college students betray their propensity for destruction of others, men and women permit the quantification and tabulation of their orgasms, and scientists lie to their subjects.

However, as sad as it is to see people voluntarily giving up their right to tell the world that some things are nobody's business but their own, it is quite another matter to have "research" done on people who are not aware that they are giving up their right to privacy.

A needy old person may, in his attempts to maintain a friendly relationship with a social worker who supplies housekeeping help for him, tell her that he goes out at night to political meetings. It is an outrage that the social worker copies this information down, adds to it from what more she learns during the friendly conversation, and then secretly turns it all over to a gerontologist who uses it and then secretly turns it into permanent government files.

How many of us have our private activities filed in this way and accessible for purposes we have never approved?

SITUATION 10: Even with the new law that gives us the right to know what the various levels of government have on file about us, we must first find if such a file exists, then where it is held, and then doggedly combat the resistance of reluctant clerks to permit us what is our right under law.

It may be argued that data about various groups are necessary in order to ascertain what the groups need and how well they are getting along in life, but it is not at all clear how doing research and collecting data on people without their full knowledge and cooperation has ever changed their lives for the better.

Nor is it any comfort to have a clerk tell us to have faith in the benevolence of those who stand guard over our files. The evidence is that, although it has been virtually impossible in the past to discover what information various government agencies keep on us, and is at present very difficult to do so, it is undoubtedly true that many institutions, businesses, and even individuals have had access to these data without our knowledge, often with devastating effect on peoples' lives.

SITUATION 11: Discussants of this situation almost invariably start from the premise that old people need "help" in adjusting productively to their age. It is obviously true that our society offers few guidelines for living as an old person. There are almost no data that can be used, by either the old or the young, as a basis for deciding what is best for old people to do with their time.

In the absence of such data, it would seem only fair, since younger adults are not obliged to submit to programing of their everyday activities by others, that old people be equally free to plan their lives in ways that suit their individual needs and desires. If they are *not* free, it is largely because lack of money captures them and imprisons them in the programs designed by community philanthropists and social workers. People with money are not likely to avail themselves of the neighborhood senior citizens' centers.

Shanas et al. and Rosenmayr suggest that a preferable alternative to organized help is family support. "All public action to give support to the aged classifies them . . . as old.[13] It is the dialectics of generally organized help to a certain group that this group becomes conscious of a certain bereavement; whereas individual and informal help and assistance based on intimacy may avoid this type of consequence: this is another reason for viewing family support as an important channel of social policy." [14]

An even more preferable alternative, I think, might be more adequate direct payments to individuals.

Maybe we ought to stop thinking in terms of "protecting" the aged, and more in terms of not interfering with their due.

Practicing New Behaviors: Simulation

You might try what a state nursing home relocation team in Pennsylvania encourages nursing home staff members to experience in preparation for moving old people from one home to another. They wear blurred glasses and surgical gloves, they put clay in their ears and cotton in their noses, all for the purpose of simulating partial loss of the senses. Walking down steps, listening to people speaking, savoring food, and even handling small pills become major problems, sources of frustration and even of danger. Perhaps, after such an experience, it would be easier to contain the annoyance at having to repeat a sentence over and over again, the impatience when someone continually slops over the liquid in a glass because he cannot see how full it is.

When you have done this, you might like to try on some new behaviors of your own, to see how they feel before you try them in real life. Role playing, for example, is a safe way to practice a variety of responses in a simulated situation. You can see how people react, first to one behavior and then to another. When you find yourself in a similar situation, on the job or socially, you then have a repertory of responses and some idea of the effects these responses have on people. You are not caught unprepared by the reality and compelled to respond on the spur of the moment. The margin for error in such behavior is obviously much greater than the possibility for error in behavior that is based on prior knowledge and experience.

You might start by taking the parts of some of the people in the situations in Exercise D and dealing in a variety of ways with the problems presented. Take the parts of old people sometimes and younger people other times. Being an old person will help you understand some of the feelings of old people in such situations; being the younger person will give you opportunity for trying behaviors you never have used before and that you have always thought you never *could* use. In role playing, you are pretty safe; no irrevocable mistakes can be made. If you don't like the consequences of a particular behavior, you can discard it and try another, until you find one you think is right.

Practicing New Behaviors: Reality

One you have examined some new behaviors in a simulated setting, you might try putting them into practice—on the job, socially, in casual contacts.

1. After watching a nurse call an old person she has just met by his first name (when she calls you, a colleague, by your last name), try accepting *your* introduction to the old person by using the same behavior you would use when you are introduced to a person your own age.

2. The next time you see an old person you already know, tell her something about yourself that you have told a younger person you have known just as long.

3. Try to break down the pattern of age separation you see where you work or play. Take a step by joining the other group, or asking the other group to join yours.

4. After listening to a physical therapist raise his voice conspicuously every time he works with an older person, point out what he's doing, and ask him if there is a medical reason for his behavior.

5. After hearing someone respond to a person with, "Isn't he marvelous? He's 75 years old!" make a point of discussing this remark with the old person after the other has left. You might start by observing, "I wonder what she has in mind when she says a thing like that."

6. Get to know adults who are living with aged parents and begin to think of the possibility that one day you will be living with an aged parent.

7. Get involved in making some changes in institutional practices:

a. Hire an older person rather than a younger when you find two applicants who seem equally qualified.

b. Get behind a movement to eliminate the mandatory retirement age where you work. This may require periodic evaluation for competency of workers of *all* ages, but incompetence is a more logical basis for retirement than age.

c. Resist the assignment of patients to rooms on the basis of age.

d. Become involved in in-service educational programing to raise consciousness regarding the existence of prejudice and discrimination against the aged. Include in the sessions people who are old and members of their families, as well as the professionals in your institution.

8. Check yourself in six months and see if your answers to the following questions indicate that your life is *not* characterized by ageism:

a. How many close friends do you have? What is the range of their ages?
b. What is your favorite pastime? Have you ever engaged in it with someone twenty or more years older (or younger) than you?
c. How many acquaintances do you have? What is the range of their ages?
d. When you are introduced to a person, how long is it before you are calling her by her given name? Does your answer depend on the status of the person? Does your answer depend on the age of the person?
e. When was the last time you said to a person twenty or more years older (or younger) than you, "Let's have lunch"?
f. When you gripe about things on the job, do you gripe only to people about your own age?
g. Have you ever double-dated with a couple twenty or more years older (or younger) than you?
h. Do you modify your language in any way when you speak to a person twenty or more years older (or younger) than you?

i. Do you believe that a person deserves "respect" just because he's older than you are?

j. Do you believe that old people need a special kind of protection?

k. Have you discussed with your parents the possibility that they may some day live with you in your home?

Helping Others To Learn

The nurse is inevitably looked to by patients and their families as a source of information and wisdom, not only about matters medical but about all kinds of problems that arise out of illness, debility, and death. Some of the discussion that follows can be useful, not only in helping the nurse to live and work more comfortably with old people, but also in helping the families of old people who are patients.

Expectations must be adjusted to fit the current reality. People who live with individuals whose senses are showing signs of deterioration, who are unable to remember many recent events, and who may also be unable to sustain a reasoning sequence may have to find resolutions to problems without the intellectual involvement of the old person. But this does not mean that all hope of a satisfying relationship must be abandoned. It is amazing what comfort and reassurance and freedom from anxiety can do even for people whose medical prognosis is hopeless. I know of one man who suffered extensive brain damage that manifested itself in aphasia. For weeks his family sat at his bedside talking to him— about the past, about the grandchildren, about happy memories and sad ones. The doctor, when he came by, insisted that there was no point in doing this. "If he's going to get better, he'll get better without all that. Don't waste your time." What he couldn't appreciate was the look in the old man's eyes as he listened, and the clasp of his hand on the hand of each family member. The old man recovered completely, and even the doctor expressed surprise at the rapidity of his recovery.

The emotional and intellectual satisfactions that might have been appropriate to the early parent-child relationship must be abandoned. The grown offspring is no longer her doting father's precious little girl, so she must not expect to be supported in every controversy, have every tantrum petted away, every birthday remembered. Perhaps these days his physical symptoms are more important to him than her current problem, and his need for peace greater than his eagerness to enter the fray on her side.

The pace of interaction with the old person must be significantly slowed. There is no sense in imposing your need to hurry on someone who simply cannot move quickly. Impatiently to push his fumbling hands from the buttons of his coat and efficiently to finish dressing him impresses on him his disability and takes the joy out of the anticipated outing. To sigh with exasperation when he cannot follow the thread of a conversation, to shout the words he cannot hear the first time, will make it clear to him that he is a troublesome burden. You don't want the kind of resigned withdrawal that so often characterizes the people in nursing homes who have been convinced that they are troublesome burdens.

The psychological space of each person in a family must be preserved.

"I'm just cutting some vegetables for the salad, Mother. It's not necessary for you to stand there and watch me. Why don't you make yourself comfortable in the living room until it's time to eat?"

"I like watching you do that."

"Yes, but it makes me nervous. I really don't want you to stand there."

"I want to be a part of everything you do."

"Are you going out tonight?"

"Yes, Dad."

"With a man or a woman?"

"A woman."

"Do I know her?"

"No."

"Why don't you bring her here sometime?"

"I will, Dad."

"When will you bring her?"

"Sometime."

"Don't you want to bring her to your home, or is it just because I'm here?"

In both these cases, the adult offspring felt pushed almost beyond endurance. The result was frequent episodes of explosive anger, recriminations that dredged up ancient resentments, hurt bewilderment, and guilt.

The story of one son who found an answer for himself may provide some guidelines for living with an aged parent—and for growing old. Our culture offers so few such guidelines that the story may sound apocryphal and the "guidelines" rejected out of hand.

John never gave much thought to his life-style until his father came to live with him. Then he suddenly realized that the style he had developed for himself since leaving his parents' home could not possibly continue. How could he bring a dinner companion home for a "nightcap" while his father slept five feet away? How could he, on the spur of the moment, accept an invitation to spend the weekend skiing, when he knew his father was waiting at home to have dinner with him? And would his father pick up the refrain he had heard since he was 19: When are you going to get married and settle down? John *knew* he didn't want to start hearing that again; he'd managed to avoid hearing it the past ten years except on holidays, when he took a trip back home.

For a while, John came home right after work. His evenings out started after dinner and ended early—alone. His weekends were devoted to shopping for groceries and "spending time with Papa." His life-style now reminded him of the years when he was in high school, and he was not happy at all.

How could he absorb his father into his home and his life and continue to enjoy the pattern he had worked out for himself? Was this at all possible, or was he just kidding himself? Did one of them have to give up, sacrifice, suffer so that the other could pick up the threads and go on as before?

John considered his father: Just who was this man he had taken into his home? What was he like? Would he make a congenial companion for a younger man? What about his political ideas? His attitude toward women? His preferences in social occasions? If this man were not his father, would he choose him for a friend?

John's answers to his own questions surprised him. He found that, when he factored out the concept "father," he saw another person that he liked, that he could enjoy, that he did not at all mind living with! So he relaxed and began to live again.

He invited friends to dinner, and his father made a fifth at the table. When his father met a charming woman, she became a sixth. When John brought a woman home with him, his father stayed discreetly in his own room, as any housemate would. Sometimes they went out together, just the two of them, to dinner and a movie. Other times his father stayed at home, pointing out that 75 was not 50.

What John found fantastically exhilarating was the realization that burst upon him one day that he was no longer carrying with him the childhood feelings of resentment and embarrassment that assailed him whenever his parents invaded his world of school or play. His father's accent fell pleasantly on his ears now; his old-fashioned good manners delighted his friends; and his interest in everything they said made him welcome in any gathering. Like many men who share a home, they lived their separate lives and came together when it suited them both.

It is true that the father needed more waiting-on, needed to be reminded to take his pills, and more than seldom observed that it was time his son married and settled down. But friendships have survived greater provocations than these, and John and his father *were* friends.

In the final analysis, old people are not a "cohort," not "the aged," not a problem to be solved. They are merely individuals grown old.

The greatest disservice done to old people is to treat those who are not impaired as if they were, depriving them of control over their own lives and reinforcing in them the negative self-concepts generated by our attitudes toward aging. Isolation, inactivity, and institutionalization contribute to the negative self-valuation of old people. When we add to this the effects of our modern technological trends that deprive old people of influence and of the opportunity to use their knowledge and skills, we not only hasten the destruction of a valuable human resource, but we set the stage for our own inevitable destruction.

Now we are taken up with the consuming concern for "death with dignity." [15]

Nurses, with their professional commitment to optimum human interaction, go beyond the merely medical objective of healing. They are the ones who, in the face of the agitation pro and con concerning euthanasia, must keep their sights on that essential humanistic commitment, even if it means resisting coming to a final decision at this time.

Taking sides on euthanasia these days is more emotionally than rationally determined, because we have not yet, as a society, faced the facts of our relationships. Either decision, to let someone die, or to make him die, is fraught with monumental danger in a society that has only just begun to struggle with its anti-humanistic attitudes and behaviors.

If a person learns he is to die shortly, he may indeed feel that his life is of no further use to him. It may, however, be possible to help him to experience this final part of his life as one in which he has much to give and to get. Are there many physicians who are at this moment in our history able to perceive the period of dying in this way? I think there are many more nurses who are at least receptive to the idea, and are willing to involve themselves in the lives of the dying patient and his family, so that this final stage of life may become a time for resolution of ancient problems and development of greater understandings. After the initial fear and anger and depression, if no decision to kill or let die is made, the patient may work through to love and hope and peace—no mean objectives at any stage of life.

Competency in decision-making is in some significant measure a function of attitudes and values. The perception and analysis of life situations are affected by what a person thinks is important, what frightens him, what repels or delights him. Thus, a white person reared to fear black people will see menace in a black person's approach, and will actually see a threatening gesture or a weapon where none exists.

Thus, an individual, fearful of growing old because he is convinced that the aged are useless (the "rolelessness" defined by some social theorists!) may be betrayed by his fear into a decision to end a life that has purpose he does not see. Thus, if the prospect of death is unreconcilably terrifying to a person, he may feel that it is better to end life as soon as medical resources are exhausted, rather than to give a patient time to come to terms with the fact of his own dying.

Thus, too, in a society like ours, where some still argue that Blacks, or Chicanos, or Puerto Ricans are less worthy of education; that Jews are less worthy of acceptance; that southern Europeans are less worthy of being Americans; that Orientals are forever outsiders—how far is it to the judgment that in this or that circumstance all of these people would be better off dead? (Didn't the Nazis propound their final solution in the name of euthanasia? Are all the Nazis among us gone?)

Even in the realm of medical knowledge, there is so much disagreement that a decision is as likely to be wrong as to be right. For example, Dr. Cecily Saunders, of St. Christopher's Hospice in London, has said that it is not necessary for the terminal patient to live with unbearable pain. With a carefully designed management program, any patient can live relatively comfortably until he dies.

At the same time, we see people suffering horrible pain.

Just what *is* possible in the management of pain? Are we giving this question the research time it deserves? Or are we so fearful of death, so defensive about failing to maintain life, that a diagnosis of terminality makes it easier to deal with the question of euthanasia than to face prolonged involvement with a dying patient?

If there is any chance at all that the remaining life is worth the suffering to the sufferers, it is the nurse who is probably in the best position to know it. Not only does she spend more time with the patient than the doctor does, and more time than family members, but the concern of nurses with the sociological and psychological bases of illness and health and their study of communication makes them more skillful at understanding the subtleties of human need and fulfillment. (The current seminars on death and dying are attended by far more nurses than physicians.) It is nurses who are in the best position to see evidences of continuing growth for patient and family, and best able to help the process along.

We can say with great confidence that the focus of our deliberations should be on encouraging optimal living (even when death is near) rather than on euthanasia. When we have really made progress in assuring the best in living for everyone, then, perhaps we can, with equal confidence, make the decisions about euthanasia.

Notes

1. Adapted from Louis E. Raths, Merrill Harmin, and Sidney B. Simon, *Values and Teaching: Working with Values in the Classroom,* Charles E. Merrill Publishing Company, Columbus, Ohio, 1966.

2. Arnold M. Rose, "Future Developments in Aging: Perspectives," reprinted from U.S. Congress Senate Hearings on Long-Range Program and Research Needs

in Aging and Related Fields, 1967, in *Perspectives in Aging, I. Research Focus,* edited and compiled by Frances G. Scott and Ruth M. Brewer, Oregon Center for Gerontology, Eugene, Oregon, 1971, pp. 7–14.

3. Gordon F. Streib, "Intergenerational Relations: Perspectives of the Two Generations of the Older Parent," *Journal of Marriage and the Family,* Vol. 27, No. 4, November, 1965, pp. 471–476.

4. Leopold Rosenmayr, "Family Relations of the Elderly," *Journal of Marriage and the Family,* November, 1968, pp. 672–680.

5. Ibid.

6. Ibid., citing Paul J. Reiss, "The Extended Kinship System: Correlates of and Attitudes on Frequency of Interaction," *Marriage and Family Living,* Vol. 24, No. 4, 1962, p. 337.

7. Rose, op. cit.

8. Ibid., quoting Geneva Mathiasen, "A New Look at the Three-Generation Family," unpublished paper presented at the 87th Annual Forum, National Conference on Social Welfare, June, 1960.

9. Rosenmayr, op. cit.

10. Ibid.

11. Bill Mandel, "What Makes Maggie Kuhn Gallop—at 69?" *The Philadelphia Inquirer,* April 27, 1975.

12. Sharon R. Curtin, *Nobody Ever Died of Old Age,* Little, Brown and Company, Boston, 1972.

13. Ethel Shanas et al., *Old People in Three Industrial Societies,* Routledge & Kegan Paul, Boston, forthcoming.

14. Rosenmayr, op. cit.

15. Charlotte Epstein, "Nursing Implications of the article by James Rachels— *Active and Passive Euthanasia,*" *Nursing Digest,* Vol. IV, No. 4, Fall, 1976, pp. 52–55.

a note on the future

If you must contemplate the future, think of yourself as the vanguard of any one of a number of possible future worlds. It is fashionable these days to do what one science fiction writer calls "grok" the future. Commissions on a national level as well as in various institutions are instructed to "dream" about the future, let their imaginations build on the current trends and indications. The results are mixed. As William Irwin Thompson says of one such "gathering of experts" called together in 1965 and 1966, "What they came up with was a fairly accurate picture of the year 1965. . . ." [1] Perhaps we, free from the constraints of fellow commission members, can break away more from the present—both frightening and forewarning ourselves. If a current trend continues, the year 2000 will have 148 older women for every older man. Given the continuation of another current trend, women will still be campaigning for equality. Since older women, unable yet to get meaningful, paid work in their own fields, will have much more time than younger women to work with politicians, consumer groups, and community activist organizations, they will be the ones who will finally become a majority among officeholders at every level. Although we will be a society led by women, we will resemble *in no way* the concept of a matriarchal society, because the women leaders will be people first, and women only for purposes of bearing children.

Because they have been members of minority groups, one would think that women—and older women, at that—would be more humanistic in their approach to the problems of government. But they will not. They will still see war as a viable solution to international problems. (One has only to see the glowing pride on the faces of some "Gold Star Mothers" to realize that women will have rationalizations for war as strong as those that men have traditionally had.)

Nor will their concern for older people or their creativity in providing for their needs rise above the current level of intermittent study and programing. Their attitude will be, "*I* made it to where I am today, let *them* make it the same way. Nobody gave *me* any handouts. *They* should have provided for their old age."

So there will be economizing on the studies and the programs, and even on the emergency financial appropriations. Perhaps it will be during the political regime of older women that there will be a revolution led by the aged.

You don't care for this vision of the future? Well, how about this one?

The age span is increasing significantly, and in the future the population will be dominated by the majority—older citizens.[2]

In the first place, it is clear that the terms of exploitation will be reversed. The elderly will no longer be second-class citizens; that role will be visited upon the young. The young will be those whom society will "put away" in custodial care homes. The aim will be to hold them in suspended animation. Some, the more promising ones genetically, will undoubtedly be cryogenically immobilized in cold storage until the elders have the quantity and quality of youth they require for replenishing their own numbers. For the elderly will suffer an attrition rate through accident, suicide, and murder; murder, of course, will become the leading cause of death, and elaborate security precautions will surround each of the aged, who will be under constant threat of attack by young people anxious to make openings that will permit them to move into the company of the elders. Of course, if birth rates too far exceed demographic replenishment needs, many of the young will have to be quietly disposed of in the future's characteristic version of euthanasia. It will only be an act of kindness to "pull the plug" on those of the young who can look forward to no useful function among the elders.

Try this vision on for size:

Old people have access to more drugs than other age groups. Most of them are legal drugs, bought over the counter or prescribed by physicians. Most of the drugs used are analgesics, tranquilizers, and sedatives— no narcotics or stimulants. Some of the aged are brought to emergency rooms suffering from drug overdose. Most of the cases appear to be accidental, the result of self-medication and the desire to experience the euphoric effect that is the side effect of some of the drugs.[3]

Can you imagine a future population of old people who, during youth, have deliberately "turned on" with a variety of drugs, including the alcohol so popular with *their* ancestors? As they get older and begin to suffer more from the various illnesses of advancing age, they add to their personal pharmacopoeia the drugs they get to treat themselves and the drugs their physicians prescribe. Eventually, our society produces a generation of old people who are almost completely out of it—living in the fuzzy, unreal world of the multidrug addict. The nation is relatively complacent about them; the attitude generally is that "They have lived their lives; what does it matter what they do now, as long as they don't do damage to anyone else?"

So, most of the old people are warehoused in reasonably comfortable facilities, where they get their drugs regularly. As a pastime, they negotiate with staff and visitors for additional drugs, and their status in the Home depends on the quantity and variety of "outside" drugs they can manage to inveigle. They do not go hungry or suffer from cold or fear the ravages of criminals. They die—quietly or raging—out of sight of anyone who might feel a personal sense of grief and loss. The country has solved the problem of the aged.[4]

> It may not be too much of a caricature to picture the year 1995 studded with retirement communes peopled by centenarian longhairs, each one with a guitar in his hand, beaded, fringed, and bathed in strobe light. The highways may well be clogged with gray-bearded hitchhikers. Dirty old men and garishly rouged Gertrude Stein-type hags could easily become society's sex symbols . . . a dominant class of elders preserving into their nineties, and many decades beyond, the life-styles, the protest movements, the arts and crafts, the communes, and the diseases of the present.

Perhaps a holocaust—nuclear warfare or pollution overload—will decimate the population and seriously affect the intellectual abilities of those who are born. The experience and intelligence of the total culture will be largely vested in older people, who already constituted 50 percent of the population in the year 2000. At first, efforts will be made to continue to scorn the superior life wisdom of the aged, but it will soon become apparent that the culture will not survive unless it is put to practical use. Gradually the elders begin to be sought out for answers to seemingly insoluble questions—just as gradually they begin to realize that they have the power to assume control. But, drawing on their knowledge of the past, and filled as they are with love for the offspring who rejected and neglected them, they develop programs for universal reeducation of the adult population and purposefully begin to institute the machinery for compulsory education.

Henceforth, adults must attend school daily for nine months of the year. The length of the school year is a touch of tradition that the old people think the younger ones need in order to reestablish lost social stability. For purposes of economy and efficiency, they will be taught in groups of forty and fifty, all of them learning expeditiously what the old person teaching has accumulated over the years. If they do not understand the practical utility of what they are being taught, they will be told, kindly but firmly, that they will understand all when they have developed the knowledge and sophistication of the old. They will be kept in school or in low-level, non-policy-making positions until they have reached the age of 60, at which time they will be admitted to the free competition of the old people's world.

The reeducation process will be most forcefully pursued with special groups made up of gerontologists, geriatrists, social workers, pediatricians, urbanologists, whites who have made a profession of studying Blacks and native Americans, the Anglos who are experts in Chicano and Puerto Rican culture. These specialists, none of whom has ever been able to solve the problems of the groups he specialized in, will have to learn the language of the ordinary person and develop an approach to their work based on the ability to communicate with those people who are their specialties.

Many futurists see a decline in industrial growth and even a zero industrial expansion. The emphasis in the future, then, will be not on money but on quality of life. Those needs that can be met by money will be provided for; the money will be allocated through one means or another. The important thing at that time will be making life better, and definitions of "better" will not rely solely on material comforts. They will involve the quality of human interaction, people relating to people in myriad helpful, caring ways. There will be no special help for the marginal or the "disadvantaged." There will be no charity for institutions and agencies deprived of financial support because of society's neglect of one group or another. All of us will give freely of ourselves and accept from others. Money will not be the important factor in the giving, because material things will be readily available for all.

In this kind of world there will be more seven-year-olds who will remember with some sadness but also with memories of great good the 75-year-old woman who had lived next door and the 80-year-old man who had lived across the street until recently. Like the seven-year-old who said to me the other day, "All our friends are dying."

Notes

1. William Irwin Thompson, *At the Edge of History,* Harper & Row, New York, 1971, p. 152.

2. Harvey Wheeler, "The Rise of the Elders—Will the World of Tomorrow Really Be Dominated by Young People?" *Saturday Review,* December 5, 1970, pp. 14–15, 42–43.

3. David M. Petersen and Charles W. Thomas, "Acute Drug Reactions Among the Elderly," *Journal of Gerontology,* Vol. 30, No. 5, September, 1975, pp. 552–556.

4. Wheeler, op. cit.

index